THE PARK AVENUE NUTRITIONIST'S PLAN

ALSO BY JANA KLAUER, M.D.

How the Rich Get Thin

THE

PARK AVENUE NUTRITIONIST'S PLAN

The No-Fail Prescription for Energy, Vitality & Weight Loss

JANA KLAUER, M.D.

ST. MARTIN'S PRESS ❧ NEW YORK

www.stmartins.com

Design by Patrice Sheridan

LIBRARY OF CONGRESS CATALOGING-IN-PUBLICATION DATA

Klauer, Jana.
    The Park Avenue nutritionist's plan : the no-fail prescription for
energy, vitality, and weight loss / Jana Klauer—1st ed.
      p. cm.
    Includes index (p. 215).
    ISBN-13: 978-0-312-37848-6
    ISBN-10: 0-312-37848-3
    1. Nutrition.   2. Physical fitness.   3. Vitality.   4. Weight loss.
5. Health.

RA784.K52 2008
613.7—dc22   2008005783

First Edition: May 2008

10 9 8 7 6 5 4 3 2 1

MEDICAL DISCLAIMER

For Gerold

CONTENTS

ACKNOWLEDGMENTS

This book comes from a desire to help people understand how certain foods, exercise, and stress management can improve their lives. The food we eat *becomes* us, in a sense. It is important to understand how different foods work within our bodies.

First, I want to thank my wonderful patients. I am privileged to know you and am moved by your trust of me. You have enriched me more than you can imagine.

Columbia University's Institute of Human Nutrition continues to offer superb courses for physicians. Notable recently is the series on the benefits of omega-3 fat on health. Richard Deckelbaum, M.D., and Sharon Akabus, R.D., Ph.D., are to be commended for getting the word out to doctors on the subject.

Martha Stewart has brought her standard of excellence to the Martha Stewart Center for Living at The Mount Sinai Hospital in New York City, which brings seniors the benefits of meditation, tai chi, walking programs, nutrition, and alternative medicine. It is a joy to see this happen and to be associated with the project.

François Payard's recipes are so perfect. I'm so grateful to be able to include them in this book.

Thank you to Richard Curtis, my trusted agent, for working out details and encouraging me. Your advice is always solid.

St. Martin's Press again gets a round of applause from me. Sally Richardson, the publisher, and Elizabeth Beier, my editor, have my unending gratitude, as do Michelle Richter and Tara Cibelli—they are just wonderful. Wendy Lewis, the book whisperer, turned around my poor words and made them user-friendly. John Murphy, head of publicity, and Colleen Schwartz worked energetically to get the word out. Sales, marketing, design, production—everyone at St. Martin's gets kudos from me. I appreciate the efforts of every single person at that remarkable company.

My trainer, Joe Masiello of Focus Integrated Fitness, saw me through the awful months of my knee injury and managed to keep the rest of my body strong. His advice on the exercise chapter was spot-on.

Shakila Rosario, the star of my office, gets a big thank-you. Your humor, poise, and gentle grace make every day a delight.

My dear husband and tango partner, Gerold, is always there for me. Thank you for it all. My children, Erika and Matthew, fill me with joy.

VITALITY, THE SOURCE OF HEALTH

*New York has a trip-hammer vitality
which drives you insane with restlessness,
if you have no inner stabilizer.*

—ARTHUR MILLER

New York is often referred to as "the city that never sleeps." New Yorkers are known for boundless energy and excitement. They are by their very nature unwilling to miss out on any of it. Fast-paced multitaskers, everyone is on their BlackBerrys 24/7. New York residents typically take less vacation time than residents of most other regions in America. The phrase "New York minute" describes New Yorkers to a tee. They don't want to wait more than a minute and can fit more into a minute in time than anyone else on the map.

My high-profile patients lead busy, hectic lives that are scheduled to the nanosecond. The result is that their energy supplies get depleted and they feel as if they are slipping into a state of total exhaustion—both physically and emotionally. New Yorkers are like the Energizer Bunny; if they keep going at a frenetic pace, 24/7, they will eventually hit a wall.

My daily routine rarely varies. I am up at 5:30 A.M. to work out for an hour, have a healthy breakfast, and then walk along Park Avenue to my office, where I review laboratory records and charts of the patients I will see throughout the day. My work is very rewarding. As a physician specializing in nutrition, daily I see people turn their lives around. Men and women from all walks of life—stockbrokers, restaurant owners, real estate developers, physicians, dentists, schoolteachers, lawyers, socialites, and even religious clergy—are patients of mine. Across the board they complain of low energy, fatigue, and sleep difficulties. But as they follow my plan, they become revived and invigorated. While cardiologists and internists can be satisfied knowing their prescriptions enable their patients to live longer, I feel like I have the added gratification of witnessing true transformations every day.

MY INSPIRATION—MAGGIE ELLA

I often tell my patients about my grandmother, Maggie Ella. She was a dynamic, energetic woman who lived her life and raised seven children on a farm. Her impact on me was immense and my memories of her are strong. She was in perpetual motion. When I stayed with her we would feed the chickens first thing in the morning. Then she did the laundry, put the clothes through the wringer, and hung them on the clothesline with wooden clothespins. And I can still remember the fresh scent of my bed linens, which my grandmother ironed after they had dried in the Texas air. We picked vegetables from the garden for dinner; I shelled peas and snapped green beans into bite-size portions. We baked bread together every other day. My grandmother caught one of her chickens, wrung its neck, plucked the feathers, and then cooked it for dinner. There was no dishwasher, except my grandmother. All pots, pans, glasses, and dishes were hand washed. The house was spotless. She did an enormous amount of physical work daily. It was tiring, I am sure, but it was a source of pride for her. She would have laughed at the idea of a personal trainer!

Maggie Ella showed me how to have a zest for life, as this is what kept her going. Even when her days were long and she had her aches and pains, her spirit never wavered. She was strong, had a positive attitude toward her life—and her health—and she lived to the ripe old age of ninety-three! Her natural energy was driven by her exuberant spirit.

WHAT IS ENERGY?

The term *energy* is widely used in various areas of life and may have many meanings ascribed to it. In science, energy is a concept that relates to the capacity of matter to perform work as the result of its motion or its position in relation to forces acting on it. Energy is sometimes used as a synonym for psychological motivation, creativity, excitement, or responsiveness. Fatigue or a lack of energy can be a result of expending chemical energy in the body or glucose and its derivatives in the brain, or a psychological condition brought on by many factors, including stress, intense emotional experiences, inadequate sleep, or an imbalance in hormones and neurotransmitters.

My patients have demanding schedules, as I do, but by reorganizing and reprioritizing their lives, they can discover new vitality. Today most people work longer hours than at any time in our history. For those reaching for the top of the pyramid, a twelve-hour workday is the norm; in fact, an eight- or ten-hour workday is considered a "light" day. But working long hours does not mean that you have to sacrifice energy.

The challenge for all of us is to make our day healthy. Make the effort to be kinder to yourself by giving your body enough sleep each night, whenever possible. Eliminate excess fat and sugar from your diet and replace them with foods that give your body fuel rather than empty, energy-zapping calories.

WHAT IS YOUR GOAL?

This is one of the first questions I ask all patients who visit my private practice. Define your goals and have a plan. Just as you have a plan in business so it must be with your health and diet.

As I wrote in my first book, *How the Rich Get Thin* (St. Martin's Press, 2005), there are *nonnegotiables* when it comes to enhancing your energy:

- Add daily aerobic exercise to your schedule no matter how busy you are.
- Include protein at every meal.
- Eliminate processed carbs.
- Eat a healthy breakfast.

In this, my second book, I will share my philosophy about how to invigorate your energy supply, reduce your stress level, improve your health, and get the rest your body needs every day. There is a difference between feeling stimulated and feeling energized. Energy comes from consistent sleep patterns, which allow your body to process food and oxygen effectively, and to rejuvenate itself in preparation for the next day's tasks—and from solid eating habits and a structured fitness routine. You need this energy to work, play, and live life to the fullest. Athletes and fitness-conscious individuals often experience a high that seems like energy but is really an adrenaline rush. Fortunately, this is a healthy type of stimulation, which comes from the body's natural stores of energy.

The more you fuel your body with what it needs to function at its best, the better it will run!

CHAPTER ONE

LET'S GET ENERGIZED!

Love is an energy which exists of itself.
It is its own value.

—THORNTON WILDER, *TIME* MAGAZINE,
FEBRUARY 3, 1958

So here you are. You have the job you always wanted. And you are really good at it. Everyone knows you are a star. You worked pretty hard to get here. But lately you just do not have the energy and drive that you once had. You are still getting all your work done, but it just isn't as much fun.

Lately you have trouble sleeping; you heard on TV about a new pill that helps you to fall asleep faster. You need to get up early and be alert at work so you consider trying the new sleeping pill. Funny, because you used to sleep like a baby, right?

You are happily married and you have always enjoyed an active sex life. Now you don't care. You are just too tired!

You think you know what the problem is. You just need to finish one of your many projects that are on your mind, such as:

- Renovating the kitchen.
- Finalizing the proposal for the merger.
- Finding a nursing home for your parents.

- Getting your children into school.
- Selling your business, or whatever.

You *think* you know how to fix the problem. Think again. You *don't* know. The reason you are reading this book is that you do not know, and you need help. The truth is you need to change your life. But it isn't nearly as scary as it sounds. Several commonsense principles combined with new scientific findings can make an enormous difference in your health and energy. Nothing is all that difficult and most of it is fun. Chances are there are just one or two factors that are out of whack in what you are doing.

Are you working at your full potential? Do you feel that you are getting the most out of life? Are your overscheduled days making you sick? If you feel you need more vigor, don't despair. I have had patients who have had debilitating symptoms for years, but eventually they have overcome this troublesome pattern of feeling unwell to get back their confidence, vitality, and energy. It is definitely possible—and if you follow my plan, it will happen to you, too.

My patient Mary is a good example of someone in need of a lifestyle adjustment. This forty-two-year-old single mother came to see me four years ago because she was dragging herself to get through each day. She was tired when she woke in the morning and required at least two cups of coffee to get going. After readying her two young boys for school and dropping them off, she went to her office. (Mary works as an editor for a major women's magazine.) She was drowsy in the afternoon and used sugary snacks from a vending machine to pep herself up. After work she rushed to pick up her children at day care, then prepared dinner, and helped with the boys' homework. She had gotten in the habit of pouring herself a glass of wine while making dinner. Lately, the number had increased steadily to two or three glasses. When Mary turned off the lights, she had trouble falling asleep and slept fitfully. As an editor, Mary was expected to present a fashionable exterior, which she did brilliantly. Her colleagues knew little of Mary's stress or challenges. Mary's lack of energy was due to the unrelenting stress of doing too much and not taking care of her basic needs.

Because appearance was an important aspect of Mary's work, she was given beautiful clothes or shopped at private sales. She knew how to put together a look. But with little time for exercise, bulges had appeared on her body and her posture was poor. Her skin was dry and more wrinkled than her age warranted.

Her laboratory work showed borderline high cholesterol and her blood pressure was also in the borderline phase. She had not yet become ill and took no medications but she was by no means in good health. If she did not change her life, illness was a given. There are many people today whose lives are as complicated, stressful, and desperate as Mary's was. It was important for Mary to get control, for herself and for her children. Clearly, she needed to make a change, but like many people, she didn't know how.

Mary needed a health makeover plan but didn't know how to find time for exercise and healthy food. Her obstacles were obvious—time and money! Working ten-hour days at the office and then taking work home—there was little time left for Mary to exercise or concentrate on food or stress reduction. I explained to her that if she wanted this to work, she must immediately forgo her evening glasses of cabernet, increase her water consumption, and begin exercising.

THREE KEY STEPS TO CHANGE

1. **Decide that you want to change.** While this may appear obvious, sometimes people think they want to change but in reality they don't want the bother of change. Change takes effort; don't underestimate this. Is the effort worth it? You decide.
2. **Identify obstacles.** Anything that could throw you off-track is an obstacle. Example: A common obstacle to eating healthfully is an environment where the best food is unavailable. Once you identify the barriers to change you can overcome them.
3. **Come up with a plan.** Once you identify the obstacles, you need to decide how you can overcome them. Example: If healthful food is unavailable, you must bring it with you. At work, this could mean packing a nutritious lunch. For a party, you could supply an alternative lighter dish.

HEALTH HOUR

Time management was at the heart of the program I designed for Mary. Without scheduling time for herself, she was compromising her health. Sacrificing time for others is a female trait. But the truth was, if Mary did not take care of herself, there would be no one left to take care of her two boys.

I asked her to identify the one time of day when she could carve out one hour. Mary stated that after her boys were tucked into bed she spent an hour sipping her wine and answering e-mails. She had just identified what would become her Health Hour.

During her Health Hour she was told to do only two things:

1. She was instructed to order her groceries for the week online. By doing so, Mary was able to free up valuable weekend time that had been spent in the grocery store.
2. Follow any one of three exercise videos I gave her. (Each exercise video was thirty to forty-five minutes in length, followed by a ten-minute stretch.)

She was to perform only these two tasks, and nothing else. While there are those who say morning exercise is best (I am one of those people), this does not mean that morning is the only time for exercise.

MAXIMUM ENERGY

While Mary worked hard to instill in her children the best nutrition with organic meats, fish, and vegetables, she paid little heed to her own nutritional needs. She started her day with large amounts of coffee and minimal food. Her days were so busy that she rarely stopped for lunch. Her dietary log revealed that she was deficient in both calcium and protein. Many women consume too little calcium, although they know they need it for their bones. Protein is also frequently neglected. The office vending machines were what she relied on at work. Mary was starving herself of nutrition and overfeeding herself with empty calories!

FOUR-POINT FOOD ENERGY PLAN

1. **Eat every four hours.** When your blood sugar drops you don't feel energetic. In evolutionary terms, our survival depends on having adequate food. Your body's metabolism slows if there are long gaps between meals and energy is conserved.
2. **Include protein at every meal and snack.** Protein keeps you from feeling hungry longer than carbohydrate or fat. Protein is essential for building and repairing cells.
3. **Drink ten glasses of water per day.** Without adequate hydration you feel tired and unenergetic. Our bodies are composed of 80 percent water. We can live for weeks without food but only a few days without water. Without adequate hydration the blood becomes thicker and cellular waste is not efficiently eliminated.
4. **Include the food power molecules:** phytochemicals and antioxidants in plants, omega-3 fats in fish, and calcium from dairy and nondairy sources. It is important to get your vitamins from natural sources because in each individual plant many vitamins are found together. The unique combinations work in synergy, providing more benefit than the isolated individual vitamins. The same holds true for the important mineral, calcium. Calcium builds strong bones, binds harmful acids in the digestive tract, and helps with fat breakdown. Calcium is more easily absorbed from natural sources and the calcium and protein found in dairy products aid in keeping weight in an optimal range. I will explain all about the food power molecules in chapter six.

Initially, it was difficult for Mary to drink the recommended amount of water. She came up with the idea of setting her computer alarm to remind herself when it was time for another glass. By the end of the week, she no longer required the reminder. She made a point of eating a nutritious breakfast and ordered a light lunch. Difficult, too, was eliminating the vending machine snack;

but because she had prepared ahead by bringing a protein snack to work, she was triumphant. Although the changes were unfamiliar to her, after a week Mary admitted that she felt "detoxified." The toxic effect of her past behavior had a numbing, addictive element in its familiarity. Once she broke free, replacing the old elements, which sapped her energy, with natural, health-enhancing new foods and behaviors, her energy began to return.

After four years, Mary has kept her basic plan. Her boys are older and are able to walk to school together. Mary's work is still time-consuming. But her evening exercise and eating plan sustain her. Her skin glows, her posture is erect, and she walks with a spring in her step. She is not overwhelmed by her busy life.

I think there are many people who, like Mary, are exhausted by the stress of doing for others. To excel as a caretaker it is vital to nurture your own health. As your energy increases you are more alive to the experience of giving of yourself. If you have ever visited an emergency room where the doctors are ending an eighteen-hour shift, you know what I mean. The physicians may be the most dedicated doctors on the planet, but after eighteen hours of high-intensity work, they are tired. Their energy has plummeted. If you visit them at the beginning of their shift, you will see an entirely different energy level. Early in the morning they are full of pep. If you are a patient, whom would you rather see? A tired and worn-out doctor or one who is engaging and energetic? With children or whoever is being cared for—everyone appreciates energy.

Your body is designed to be energetic. If it is not energetic, you need to find out why!

ENERGY SELF-ASSESSMENT

1. Are you very sleepy or do you doze off in the afternoon?
2. Do you use caffeine to perk yourself up during the day?
3. Do you spend the weekends "catching up" on your sleep?
4. Do you exercise?
5. Do you rely on empty calories to give yourself energy?
6. Do you sleep soundly? How many hours do you sleep continuously?
7. Do you require medication for sleep? Is it impossible for you to sleep without it?

8. Do you have joy in your life?
9. Do you fall behind in your work? Do you find yourself struggling to keep up with the pace of your job?
10. Have you lost or gained weight unintentionally within the past year?

If you answer "yes" to any question other than 4, 6, and 8,—you need some help! You don't have to feel the way you do. That's the good news. Being tired is a way for our bodies to tell us that we are doing too much. It is normal to feel exhausted after an episode of intense physical activity. It is abnormal to feel chronically exhausted; you should be evaluated by your physician. After you see your doctor to rule out a metabolic reason for your energy lag, you need to address the issue.

Amazingly, the most frequent cause of lack of energy is bad habits. That is both good and bad news: good, because we can fix it, and bad, because fixing it requires changing ingrained habits.

CHAPTER TWO

THREE BAD HABITS AND HOW TO BREAK THEM

Imagine if you could stop a disease from developing within your own body. Imagine halting it in the very early stages, before the devastating effects are felt. Wouldn't it be grand? In fact, if that were possible, it is difficult to see why anyone would not do so. But the simple fact is we can prevent approximately 75 to 80 percent of all illnesses just by changing poor habits.

After years of talking to patients about their lives and diets I have pinpointed the top three bad habits that drain health and energy.

1. Eating foods that cause an inflammatory response in the body
2. Constant dieting
3. Insufficient physical exercise

The unfortunate fact is that the majority of people who are guilty of these bad habits really believe that they are living their lives in a healthy manner!

BAD HABIT #1: INFLAMMATION NATION

Inflammation is the body's way of fighting off infection.

In medical school we were taught to recognize the classic signs of inflammation: *rubor, turgor, calor,* and *dolor.* Translating the Latin gives us *redness, swelling, heat,* and *pain.*

When bacteria enter our bodies, a remarkably orchestrated immune response occurs. First, blood flow to the area increases causing redness (*rubor*) and heat (*calor*). The capillaries to the area become "leaky," allowing the white blood cells to exit the circulation and surround the infection, causing swelling (*turgor*). The white blood cells are not only kamikaze fighters, sacrificing themselves to kill the infection, but they are also messengers, sending chemical signals of the danger to surrounding cells. They produce substance P, causing pain (*dolor*).

Inflammation has enabled us to survive the innumerable bacteria we are exposed to in our lifetimes. In a sense, inflammation is a survival mechanism. So, you may ask, how is inflammation "bad" for us? The protection given by inflammation is in defending the body against invading bacteria or viruses. The protective inflammation, described by the Latin phrase, is acute inflammation. It stops when the infection is defeated.

But chronic inflammation is a whole other ball game. Chronic inflammation is a persistent state and is not limited in time. It harms the body—much of the harm is from the white blood cell production of chemical signals, or prostaglandins. Autoimmune diseases such as rheumatoid arthritis, lupus, type I diabetes, and scleroderma are examples of chronic inflammation. The joints, lungs, esophagus, heart, kidneys, skin, and virtually every organ system are affected by the inflammatory proteins. Autoimmune diseases are not the only times when chronic inflammation is present. Chronic inflammation is most commonly found in individuals who believe they are fine, except for the extra weight that's around their middle.

Belly fat actually causes inflammation. It contains types of cells called macrophages, which under normal conditions are Pac-Man–like cells cleaning up debris. But belly fat macrophages pump out inflammatory chemicals that attract the white blood cells and activate them to send out inflammatory proteins. The fat cells themselves are bigger and churn out inflammatory signals. The chronic state of inflammation raises the risk for blood clots, high blood pressure, diabetes, cardiovascular disease, and cancers of the pancreas, gall-bladder, colon, breast, and prostate. Chronic inflammation robs the body of energy.

Many people do not appreciate how their diets can lead to an inflammatory state. We can measure the degree of inflammation with laboratory blood tests that measure the levels of C-reactive protein. The chemicals of inflammation are produced from fats we eat. Trans fat and saturated fat increase inflammatory proteins and cause weight gain. Sugar causes inflammation also. American and British diets, particularly snack foods, set the stage for an inflammatory state. The marketing of the foods compounds the problem because some of the foods would seem to benefit our health.

For example: look at high-sugar yogurts. I was recently on a plane where the so-called "healthy option" for breakfast was fruit (melon, grapes, and pineapple) with a container of fat-free yogurt. Reading the yogurt label showed the first ingredient to be pasteurized skim milk, the second ingredient was sugar, and the third was high-fructose corn syrup. That doesn't sound very healthy at all. Later the flight attendant offered passengers a choice of greasy croissants or sugary Danish pastries, just to make matters worse.

The overconsumption of sugar is problematic because we all love sweetness. It has been hypothesized that the desire for sweets evolved as a means for prehistoric man to survive. Berries and edible roots are sweet but the poisonous alkaloids are bitter. Back in the caveman days, those who found the berries got a healthy boost of energy and survived. Cavemen who ate the alkaloids died. Thus, the genetic drive for sweetness was selected and endures. Maternal milk is sweet. Babies do not like bitter or sour foods.

We are so programmed to like sweetness that we call our lovers "sweetheart." Sweetness is endearing to us. The big problem nowadays is we have this innate liking of sweets and we are surrounded by sweet food. Doughnuts at the coffee shop and then coffee cake during the morning meeting; we might have a healthy lunch but when the afternoon energy lag sets in, there is always the candy machine down the hall. What about a soda with some sugar and caffeine to help pep us up in the afternoon? After dinner we allow ourselves a bowl of ice cream with (only) one cookie. I do not think that I am overstating the case, either. The day just described is more than one cup of sugar. That is more than the cavemen had to deal with in their entire life span!

THE MODERN DIET

In prehistoric times, humans had a very different diet. Grains that were consumed were small and difficult to harvest. Wild grains were hard to digest without grinding and cooking. Stone mortars and bowls first appeared in the Upper Paleolithic period (forty thousand to twelve thousand years ago). Grain seems to have played a minor role in early prehistoric time.

Before the Industrial Revolution, all grain was ground with the use of stone milling tools and contained the complete grain—bran, germ, and endosperm. In the nineteenth century, with the invention of mechanized steel rollers and sifting devices, we began our consumption of overly refined flour devoid of the nutritional value that was present in the whole grain. The flour that we now use is a recent invention of the last two hundred years.

Refined flour has the outer bran (with fiber) and germ (with vitamins) removed. Refined flour contains only the endosperm, which is starch. The reason this is done boils down to economics. Bread requires the elasticity of gluten to rise; bran interferes with the strands of gluten, complicating the rising of a loaf. And because the germ contains healthy unsaturated fat, which can become rancid, whole grains have a shorter shelf life than refined grains. Additionally, after years of being exposed to refined flour products, we have come to accept them as the norm. We have developed a "taste" for these foods. This in turn spurs the marketplace to produce more and more refined and overly processed foods. Starchy foods, which are composed of chains of sugars, are rapidly digested. We are not satisfied by eating them and become hungry quickly.

Refined sugar is a relatively new invention. Today we consume 155 pounds of sugar per person per year!

Crystallized sugar first appeared in India about 500 B.C. Honey is a natural sweetener that varied by season. Not only have we consumed increasing amounts of sugar, but the form of the sweetening has changed. It is not table sugar, or sucrose, that we find in most of our foods, but high-fructose corn syrup. The rise in obesity directly parallels our consumption of high-fructose corn syrup. Since 1970, when it was first introduced, its use has risen 1,000 percent. Today high-fructose corn syrup is used to sweeten most sweetened sodas and processed foods.

New research has found evidence that sodas sweetened with high-fructose corn syrup may contribute to the development of diabetes, particularly in children. Chemical tests of eleven different carbonated soft drinks containing high-fructose corn syrup found high levels of reactive carbonyl molecules believed to cause potential tissue damage.[1] The carbonyl groups are formed when carbonation causes fructose molecules to become unstable. The dangerous and highly reactive molecules can then cause oxidative damage. More research will determine if this is indeed the mechanism whereby high-fructose corn syrup in carbonated drinks harms us, but it is evident that our high consumption of the sweetener is worrisome.

Additional concern about fructose consumption is raised by the fact that of all the simple sugars, fructose is the only one that raises the level of uric acid within the body. Because uric acid is an inhibitor of nitric oxide, which allows blood vessels to dilate, fructose causes the vessels to constrict, leading to the elevation of blood pressure. The abundant use of fructose in processed foods may account for the increasing prevalence of hypertension seen in children and teens today.[2]

Besides adding pounds to body weight and raising the risk for disease, the inflammatory state drains your energy. Instead of being energetic and vital you are exhausted. The inflammatory habit saps your strength. Just as you would feel lethargic during an acute inflammatory response produced by an infection, with chronic inflammation you are persistently tired.

Overconsumption of high-fat and high-sugar foods has an *addictive* quality. These foods cause the release of dopamine, the neurotransmitter associated with sensual gratification. Alcohol, drugs, and food activate a region of the brain associated with pleasure, the hippocampus. Today, inflammatory food would appear to be the number one substance of abuse.

ARE YOU A JUNK FOOD ADDICT?

To find out if you are addicted to junk food, take the CAGE test. A psychiatric screening test for alcoholism, CAGE evaluates the strength of cravings. The test works just as well for overdependence on junk food as it does for alcohol.

I.   Have you ever felt the need to *Cut* down on your drinking (or eating)? Just as people who are drinking too much are aware that they are, those who are overdoing it with food know it; the problem with both is lack of control.

2. Have you ever been *Annoyed* by criticism of your drinking (or eating)? Alcoholics do not like to be reminded they are overconsuming; those who overconsume food feel the same. In both cases, the reason is overattachment to the substance of abuse.

3. Do you feel *Guilty* about your drinking (or eating)? Guilt occurs because the addict can see the damage that is occurring.

4. Have you ever felt the need for an *Eye-opener*? Just as an alcoholic has an early-morning drink, a food addict might have a food craving when he or she gets up in the morning.

If you answered "yes" to more than two questions, you may have an addiction to junk food.

PRACTICAL PORTION CONTROL

Americans seem to have lost their ability to judge a reasonable serving size. Everywhere we go, from fast food emporiums to fine dining establishments, they are serving bigger portions. The more food people have in front of them, the more they will eat. The more refined sugar you consume, the less energy you will have.

I show my patients how to wean themselves from large servings and train themselves to eat reasonable amounts without having to weigh and measure everything they put in their mouths. Portion distortion has supersized American waistlines. Twenty years ago the average adult ate almost 1,000 calories fewer than today.

Snack-size baggies: These hold about 1 cup fully packed, and about ¾ cup loosely packed carrots, cubed low-fat omega-3 enriched cheese, celery sticks, red grapes, or grape tomatoes.

Whole-grain pita bread: This is a great way to portion your sandwiches if you fill half of each pocket with raw vegetables (lettuce, tomatoes, cucumbers), then add some protein, such as grilled chicken, roasted turkey, low-fat cheese, or lean ham.

TIPS FOR EATING OUT

- Don't go to restaurants (or grocery stores) when you're starving!
- Share your meal or entrée with a companion, and order extra salads so both of you get something green.
- Cut your entrée in half and take home a doggy bag to enjoy the rest of the meal the next day.
- Inquire how the food is prepared. What type of oil is used? Don't be shy. If an entrée is not prepared in a healthful way, speak up. You are paying for the food and you deserve to have what you ask for; request a green vegetable as a substitute for a potato.

The inflammation habit attacks the brain through addiction and the body through inflammatory proteins. It robs us of vital energy.

BAD HABIT #2: THE DIETING HABIT

From time to time, the majority of us have gone on a diet. It is normal behavior in our land of abundance. But there are people who abnormally schedule their lives around unnatural eating clusters. There are several variations of the dieting habit, but the most common are "save and splurge" and "wait until dark."

SAVE AND SPLURGE—Many people have what I like to call a "save and splurge" attitude toward food. They eat anything and everything in sight at a big occasion, followed up with a day or two of severely limiting food. The problem with this eating style is the focus is solely on weight gain, without regard to nutrition. On the positive side, the person is watching their weight, but unfortunately, not giving their body what it needs for good health. Just because the scale has good news for you doesn't necessarily mean you are doing the best you can. Going for days without food to fit into a bikini on spring break is a strategy used by high school and college girls. You cannot think or perform at your highest level if you are undernourished!

There is a recognized syndrome of the effect of severely restricted food in young women who exercise. The Female Athletic Triad consists of disordered eating, loss of the menstrual period, and osteoporosis. Seen in sports that prize a slim body—gymnastics, ballet, diving, swimming, or ice skating—the syndrome illustrates the harm of severe caloric restriction on metabolism. Symptoms of the syndrome are weight loss, fatigue, low blood pressure and heart rate, hair loss, and stress fractures. This dangerous diet and exercise regimen has lasting effects as peak bone mass is compromised.

Depriving the body of food slows metabolism. Eating fewer than a thousand calories per day lowers metabolism by 10 to 15 percent. The body perceives this as starvation. In evolutionary terms, energy was conserved when food was scarce to allow for survival. Our ancestors faced famine during winter, droughts, and times of migration. Their bodies were forced to develop adaptations to cope with lack of food. What are the adaptations? Unnecessary physical activity decreases, thermogenesis (the body's natural heat production) is curtailed, and the muscle protein is broken down for energy. Because energy is limited, nonessential repairs are halted—your skin will appear dull and your hair will fall out. Fertility drops.

The dieting habit is counterproductive because of two facts:

1. The new number on the scale represents loss of both muscle and fat. Losing muscle is a bad idea because muscle mass determines resting metabolic rate. Example: Your clothes have become a tiny bit too snug so you hop on the scale and find that you have gained ten pounds! You decide to get it off quickly with the grapefruit diet or the chicken soup diet or whatever crazy plan promises the fastest result. Guess what? You succeed! But the only problem is you have lost some muscle mass in the process. The scale says the right number, but your body doesn't look as fabulous as you had hoped.

2. The lower metabolism caused by loss of muscle mass means that weight is easily regained and is harder to lose.

As we get older and less active, we need less food to live on. After age thirty our metabolism drops 5 percent per decade. Up until our mid-twenties our bodies are involved in the processes of growth and maturation; we reach our peak height, peak bone density, and peak muscle mass. We reach sexual maturity as well. Growth and maturation require large numbers of calories, and we become accustomed to eating more. Unfortunately, our eating patterns are pretty well set by the time we reach adulthood. These eating patterns cause weight gain later in life, so we diet. The trouble with a diet is that it is something you do temporarily to try to get the weight off. When the diet is over, the pounds roll back because you have not really changed your habits.

A change in attitude is the first step to a change in lifestyle. Permanent success takes retraining yourself about food and nutrition. The goal is to maintain muscle and bone mass and to keep body fat at a reasonable level. Try to think of food as fuel. Realize that the food you consume has immediate and long-term effects.

Luisa is a shoe designer who visited me with the complaint that in addition to feeling jet-lagged constantly, she was gaining weight. She made frequent trips back and forth between Italy and New York, often as many as four or five per month. Because she had followed the same schedule for the last ten years she just could not understand why she was feeling so lethargic. Her lab work was fine and did not indicate that a serious illness was the cause of her problems. She was not anemic, her thyroid status was within the normal range, and even her cholesterol profile was good. But during her physical examination I noted that she had indeed gained about twelve pounds. All else was normal. When we discussed her life, she told me her family in Italy had worked in the shoe business for generations and the company that she now headed had been started by her grandfather. Within the past year she had been phased in as her father retired. Her family was loved in both the world of fashion and politics in Italy. For a woman to take over was quite extraordinary. Because she wanted to do well and be accepted Luisa had set up a grueling schedule for herself. She dined out nightly with her business contacts in Italy, having dinners that lasted well into the evening. Her father was known for his gregarious, hospitable style—he was her role model. But what she neglected to factor in was that her father did not commute back and forth from New York City. He lived in Milan, near his factory and associates. Luisa spent a week in Italy and then returned to oversee her New York office. At the dinners in Italy, Luisa ate her fill of the delicious pasta and drank wonderful wines. But when she returned to New York (a few pounds heavier) she went on what she termed "the espresso diet," consuming only espresso and water during the day and a light dinner in the evening. Why was Luisa gaining weight and feeling lethargic? By starving herself all day Luisa caused her blood glucose to fall, leaving her tired and unenergetic. Her strategy of drinking espresso provided only a temporary jolt. The caffeine caused a surge of epinephrine that increased the heart rate and mental concentration. Epinephrine speeds up metabolism temporarily. The problem is your body receives no nutrition. You are running on empty. Sure, the body breaks down fat, which is what Luisa wanted. But muscle is also catabolized during starvation. Because muscle is an active tissue responsible for calorie burning during exercise, having less muscle means fewer calories can be burned off. When the pattern occurs often, as in Luisa's case, more and more muscle is consumed and losing weight becomes progressively harder.

WAIT UNTIL DARK—This is a common strategy of New York socialites. If you eliminate breakfast (with the possible exception of an espresso) and lunch, thereby saving all calories for dinner, it should be obvious to all that energy will suffer. Blood sugar bottoms out during the day and you feel tired and unenergetic. The large meal at night stresses the pancreas by causing a massive outpouring of insulin (a storage hormone). Large meals at night have been linked to reflux disease, a condition that is becoming increasingly prevalent. If the large meal includes alcohol or chocolate, the risk for reflux is heightened. You will feel your best if you schedule eating at approximately four-hour intervals. It takes about four hours to digest a meal, so four hours works for most people. We feed our infants on a four-hour schedule, so baby yourself and eat on a regular schedule.

Let's look at Miguel. Miguel, age thirty-seven, was a successful banker in Mexico, who first came to my office on one of his monthly business trips to

New York. He was a devoted family man, happily married with three small children. He visited me for help in overcoming jet lag from his constant travel to the United States and Europe. Miguel worried that there might be something seriously wrong with him because he was constantly tired. Additionally, even though he said he ate very little, Miguel was gaining weight. He told me that the best part of the day was when his small children came into the bedroom in the morning to wake him. After this magical start to the day, Miguel read the newspaper at the breakfast table while his children ate. Miguel usually ate a small breakfast of two cups of strong coffee and a roll with butter and jam. He skipped lunch unless he was dining with business associates. As the custom in Mexico is for a late dinner, he dined at home with his family. He went to bed at midnight and got up at 7 A.M. to play with his children before heading to his office.

When he traveled, Miguel's schedule was much less predictable. He often was out the door at 6:30 or 7 A.M., and his schedule included dinner meetings with a few bottles of good wine. Miguel had not exercised since he was in college, other than an occasional swim or game of tennis. However, he volunteered that his home in Mexico contained a full gym, which was used only by his wife. His Upper East Side apartment complex had a gym also, but he claimed that he used up all of his energy with his work and had no time to exercise!

Obviously, Miguel needed to eat nutritious foods and add exercise to his life, yet he was sacrificing himself for his work. One of the reasons why so many individuals I have met do this is that they are so driven and view exercise as "recreation" and a "distraction" from what really matters—work. Miguel agreed this was the case.

Lifestyle factors catch up with us in our thirties. I gave Miguel the following advice to follow for one month:

- Avoid the packaged airline food. Plan on eating a meal before departure, but have nothing during the flight except water. Carry an apple or a small bag of nuts or my protein bar to substitute for the airline meal.
- Add protein for breakfast. His children had free-range eggs every

morning from the family farm, so Miguel agreed this would be ideal.

- Stop skipping meals.
- Go for a walk daily. I did not give him a time limit for the walk but advised him to be consistent. Treat it as a new job.

After one month Miguel came in and had religiously followed all my advice. He was in the midst of an enormous financial deal, requiring even longer hours and more time away from his family, yet his energy was much better than before. He noted his sleep was deeper and he did not feel as stressed, although his responsibilities were huge. He felt healthier.

Are you like Miguel? Are you working to extremes? Perhaps a good way for you to view healthy behaviors is to treat this as your new job. Stop complaining about how tough it all is and do your job! The famous New Yorker Woody Allen once said, "Eighty percent of life is just showing up." Start showing up for your health job.

Both of the dieting strategies of "save and splurge" or "wait until dark" slow down metabolism. Limit your calories and your energy will suffer. Your resting metabolic rate (RMR) is roughly ten times your weight. RMR can be measured directly and it is dependent on weight, age, and sex. Resting metabolic rate means the calories you require for metabolism: breathing, circulating blood, maintaining blood pressure, digestion, etc. The RMR is the calories that you require when you sit quietly; when you start to move you add to the number. (Example: My weight is 130 pounds and my RMR is about 1,300. When I run for an hour I add 400 calories to the number.)

If you limit your calories to a number less than the metabolic rate, your metabolism begins to slow. You do not feel energetic; in fact, you feel sleepier and less alert. Your body responds with an attempt to conserve energy. It may not even be apparent to you. You subconsciously slow down energy expenditure by sleeping a few minutes longer, walking less, and not giving your best effort to exercise. Your activity is compromised because your metabolism is compromised.

Metabolic chambers are laboratory environments that accurately measure caloric expenditure by monitoring the amount of CO_2 produced. Metabolic chambers are located in research facilities and are extremely expensive to operate. But the metabolic chamber is the most accurate way of measuring exactly how many calories are being used. When an individual is severely limited in calories, studies done in the metabolic chamber show they move less than when given adequate calories.

BREAK BAD HABIT #2—Diets don't work because "going on a diet" is a time-limited behavior without regard to nutritional needs. If you are hungry and energy-depleted, chances are you are on a diet. Inevitably, you will break the diet. You will overeat and gain back the weight you lost.

What you eat is important. If your only fuel is empty calories that are quickly metabolized your energy will lag. You want nutritious, slowly metabolized energy that lasts. This will be supplied by protein and power molecules.

BAD HABIT #3: THE INACTIVITY HABIT

BREAK BAD HABIT #3—*Everyone can benefit from making physical exercise a priority.*

I have heard just about all the excuses that exist for not exercising, and that is what they are—excuses. It is not about losing weight or looking like a movie star but using the body as it is designed. We are the product of thousands of years of evolution. During those years we survived because we were active: running from danger, chasing prey, looking for food, tilling the soil, doing daily physical work. It is only in the past few hundred years, since the Industrial Revolution, that our lives have become sedentary.

The reason our lives are longer now is due to the advances in medicine, not because we are becoming healthier on our own. Inactivity causes disease. When we do not move we are encouraging fat storage and an inflammatory state. When sedentary individuals begin a regular exercise program, weight is lost more from the abdomen and the markers in the blood of chronic inflammation begin to decrease. Just by exercising you can help reduce or prevent inflammation!

Bad habits are tough to change but the reward is a happier and more energetic life. I will give you the tools to make the change in the chapter on exercise.

CHAPTER THREE

ENERGY BOOSTERS: OMEGA-3, PROTEIN, AND CALCIUM

Of all natural forces, vitality is the incommunicable one. Vitality never "takes." You have it or you haven't it, like health or brown eyes or a baritone voice.

—F. SCOTT FITZGERALD

Everyone can and should understand the basic principles of good nutrition. Simply stated, there are three food groups:

1. Carbohydrate
2. Protein
3. Fat

Any food you might be interested in will fall into one of those groups; some will fall into more than one. Carbohydrate comes from plants, protein comes from animals, and fats come from both plants and animals. Let's take an example of cereal: It comes from grain, a carbohydrate. Cereal has little protein or fat. Cereal falls into the category of carbohydrate. If the cereal is made from whole grain it will be a good source of fiber, as well. What about the milk you put on your cereal? Milk is a source of animal protein, usually about ten grams per glass of milk. But animal protein is always accompanied by saturated fat; a glass of regular milk (3.5 percent fat) contains approximately 8g fat, two percent milk contains 4g, I percent contains 2g, and skim milk is fat-free. Drink skim milk or one percent. How about berries with your cereal? What food group are they? Are they carbohydrate, protein, or fat?

Start with ½ cup of whole grain cereal (carbs and small amount of fat)

Add skim milk (carbs and protein)

Add ½ cup of blueberries (carbs)

———————————————————

Carbs + Protein + Fat

Some foods are a combination of carbohydrate plus protein (legumes), carbohydrate plus fat (vegetables), or protein plus fat, and some foods can even be a combination of all three.

CARBOHYDRATE

The large carbohydrate family is ubiquitous in nature. All plants contain carbohydrate naturally.

WHOLE GRAINS

Every grain has an outer shell of fiber that is the *bran*. The interior contains the *germ*, which contains all the vitamins and minerals in the grain. The rest of the grain is composed of *endosperm*. Endosperm is the starch, which serves as an energy reservoir so that the germ can grow into a plant. When a grain is refined, the bran coating and the germ are taken away, leaving only the starchy endosperm. Basically, this process removes all the vitamins and fiber. Enriched grains contain four of the vitamin B complex vitamins (riboflavin, folate, B_6, B_{12}), and the mineral iron. So, do that math. They took away eleven, and they put back five, so you are still missing six vitamins and all the fiber!

Grain is composed mainly of carbohydrate, but the quantity varies according to the type of grain. Carbohydrate accounts for 65 to 90 percent of the calorie content of grain. Protein usually accounts for 7 to 15 percent of the calories and the fat content, contained wholly within the germ, makes up the remainder of the calories. Grain does not contain any saturated fat or cholesterol, and is a rich source of protein, but the protein lacks some of the essential amino acids that are obtained only from animal sources. Whole grain is loaded with vitamins, fiber, and minerals, especially in the bran and germ, but these components are removed when producing refined flour. The bran is also loaded with insoluble fiber, important for digestive health, and soluble fiber, which helps to lower the cholesterol level in the blood. When whole grain and whole grain products are combined with a balanced diet, they are one of the most important foods for providing proper nutrition. But refined grain is quickly digested, raising blood sugar and insulin levels. You feel full initially but soon you feel even hungrier, and tired. How will you know if the grain is refined or whole? Read the label.

Wheat is the main grain grown in the United States and most bread and cereals contain wheat. Make it a point to read the label to be sure you are buying whole wheat. Do not be fooled by healthy sounding words: "organic wheat flour," "enriched wheat flour," and "vitamin-rich wheat flour"—all are *refined* wheat flour. Look for whole wheat as an ingredient. If the label doesn't say whole wheat, it is refined wheat. Whole wheat contains good amounts of fiber and anti-inflammatory nutrients, such as selenium, zinc, and folate. See Appendix, page 191: Nutritional Components of Grains.

FRUIT AND VEGETABLES

Fruit and vegetables contain mainly carbohydrate. But they differ from grain in that their water content is higher and their starch content is lower. The major difference between grain and fruit and vegetables is shelf life. Grain has a long shelf life and represents storage energy whereas most fruit and vegetables are perishable, requiring refrigeration.

Fruit contains more sugar than most vegetables and has on average a hundred calories per individual fruit. The sugar that fruit contains is fructose; this is important because fructose is metabolized differently than sucrose, or table sugar. Table sugar, because it is quickly absorbed from the digestive tract, immediately raises the blood glucose. When fructose is consumed it does not result in an immediate rise in blood glucose; rather, blood glucose rises gently because fructose is metabolized through the liver. You experience this as a more sustained energy rather than a sugar high. The fiber content in fruit modulates digestion, as high-fiber foods are processed more slowly. Fruit is sweet but it is metabolized slowly.

THE GLYCEMIC INDEX

The glycemic index gives an idea of how rapidly a carbohydrate can raise blood sugar. The glycemic index rates foods as low (fifty-five and under), medium (fifty-six to sixty-nine), and high (seventy and above). Pure glucose is used as a reference point at one hundred on the glycemic index. Interestingly, while it was initially thought that it was simple sugars that raised the blood glucose, now we know that starchy foods can have an even greater impact. Baked potatos, white bread, and popcorn are all higher on the glycemic index than a Snickers bar!

Interestingly, the particle size of foods affects their glycemic index. For example, the glycemic index of a one-inch cube of potato can increase by 25 percent just by mashing the potato. Blood sugar rises faster because mashing the potato increases surface area accessible to digestive enzymes. Apples and applesauce behave the same way.

Processing of food changes its glycemic index. Starch exists in carbohydrate foods in the form of large granules. When the granules are disturbed through processing, more become available for hydrolysis. Grinding, pressing, and even the act of chewing disrupt the granules and increase the glycemic index. As a general rule of thumb, processing food raises the glycemic index.

WHO SHOULD USE THE GLYCEMIC INDEX?—Diabetes or insulin resistance, polycystic ovarian syndrome, or abdominal weight gain are conditions with insulin imbalance and inflammation. Each of the conditions is made worse by excessive release of insulin. Eating foods with high-glycemic numbers adds fuel to the inflammatory fire. In fact individuals with these conditions may be given medications that help lower the insulin. Consuming high-glycemic foods works against the medications that may have been prescribed to treat the diseases. The glycemic index gives you information that you need in deciding whether or not to eat a particular food.

But because the glycemic index of any food is variable and is affected by processing, cooking, ripening, and physical form, the glycemic index doesn't tell the whole story. It is wise to understand the glycemic index—it is useful in understanding the response to a given food. Keep in mind that it is variable. See Appendix, page 198: Glycemic Index for Carbohydrate.

You also need to consider the foods that are eaten with the carbohydrate, as they too will affect blood glucose. The idea of taking into account the total amount of food and not just an isolated food is referred to as the glycemic load.

> Basically it boils down to this: By combining a high-glycemic food like a banana with a low-glycemic food like a container of cottage cheese, your blood sugar will not spike.

Our prehistoric diet consisted of a wide variety of plants, fruit, nuts, and over a hundred species of animals, fish, and insects—it was a low-glycemic diet. We did not eat corn, potatoes, or grain until agriculture was invented about ten thousand years ago. The significance of our prehistoric diet was that our digestive system evolved without having to cope with large swings in blood glucose and insulin. High-sugar foods include foods that are not thought of as "sweet"—potatoes, corn, and refined bread. Do you know that a baked potato has more free sugar than actual table sugar? Potato is starch, made up of sugar molecules linked together, whereas table sugar—sucrose—is composed of two simple sugars, glucose and fructose. Because fructose is metabolized through the liver, blood sugar does not rise as dramatically after eating table sugar as it does after eating a baked potato.

The problem with high-sugar, starchy foods is that large amounts of insulin are released, forcing the body into "storage mode." Next blood sugar plummets and you are hungry again.

Vegetables are usually low on the glycemic index because they do not have as much sugar. They are also lower in calories. Include fresh vegetables in every meal. In fact, I suggest building your meals around vegetables. Aim for lots of color as each color in nature offers different benefits. Make use of herbs to liven taste. I really do not believe it is possible to overeat vegetables!

BENEFITS OF VEGETABLES:

- Low in calories
- Low in fat (and the fat they contain is good for you)
- High in power molecules
- High in fiber
- High in vitamins and minerals

PROTEIN

Protein helps to build and repair cells. Our bodies are in a constant state of evolution. Did you know that muscles renew themselves every three months? This occurs whether you exercise or not, by the way. If you exercise an even more vigorous renewal occurs. Our skeletal bones are in a constant state of re-modeling. Our digestive system replaces cells almost weekly. In the repair process we recycle protein that is already present but also we require a constant supply.

Carbohydrate is unable to repair cells because it does not contain the molecule nitrogen. Nitrogen is found exclusively in protein. Carbohydrate and protein can be metabolized into fat. Carbohydrate and fat cannot be converted to protein; therefore we must consume it.

In nature, protein comes with fat. The egg presents a unique situation where the two are neatly separated: the yolk has the fat and the white is pure protein. In fact, the egg white is the only pure protein in nature. Sources for protein include eggs, dairy products, fish, poultry, meat, and plant protein found mainly in legumes. In my practice a frequently encountered pattern is a diet high in carbohydrate and low in protein and the mineral calcium. The usual complaint is lack of energy and lethargy. But the most concerning aspect of the picture is that it is often seen as an attempt to control calories. The truth is that protein is digested more slowly than carbohydrate, thus allowing you to feel full longer, thus saving calories.

Jane was a forty-year-old woman who worked as a freelance stylist in New York City. She traveled frequently to Asia and Europe as part of her work. When she initially came in, it was difficult to envision her keeping up with the hectic schedule that she described. I noticed her dry skin, thinning hair, and how tired she seemed. She appeared sleep-deprived and had fallen asleep sitting in my waiting room. Her diet recall revealed: Breakfast: 8 A.M. Two cups of coffee and a biscotti or instant oatmeal with water. Lunch: 2 P.M. Salad with iced tea. Dinner: 10 P.M. One martini followed by a salad, pasta primavera, and two glasses of wine. When she got home from her date, she had a frozen diet ice cream bar.

Based on her weight Jane's daily protein requirement was 70g but Jane had only given herself approximately 5g protein for the entire day! Jane was worried too about her expanding waistline. Because she exercised regularly and watched her calories, she could not understand why her waist had grown. As I explained to Jane, exercise and calories are important but they are not the whole story. You must give yourself adequate nutrition. When I reviewed her laboratory results I noted that her albumin was low. Serum albumin is a marker for general nutrition and a clear indication of protein deficiency. Assessing her body composition, I found she had little muscle mass or sarcopenia. Additionally, she was mildly anemic. No wonder Jane felt terrible—she was starved for nutrition! Even though Jane had not experienced menopause, I ordered a bone density measurement because I felt she was at risk. The bone density test revealed osteopenia, a risk for osteoporosis. The low protein and absence of calcium in her diet meant her bones were deteriorating. She had the bone mass of a sixty-year-old woman!

I encouraged Jane to start her day with my Everyday Nutrition shake, giving her 20g protein, 400mg calcium, and 700mg omega-3 fat.

I told her to stop her habit of skipping meals and advised her to have a protein-rich snack in the afternoon, and to include high-quality protein at both lunch and dinner. What I recommended to Jane had more calories than Jane was accustomed to eating, but after one month Jane lost two inches from her waist because her metabolism was not being compromised by poor nutrition. She ate the foods that her body required, not empty calories. She appeared livelier and her skin was less dry. Jane is representative of many women who attempt to control their weight by limiting their calories and neglecting nutrition.

TOP TIPS FOR GETTING YOUR PROTEIN

- Add cooked egg whites to all main-course salads. Egg white is the only naturally occuring 100 percent protein.
- Eat one or two omega-3 eggs for breakfast.
- Eat a minimum of two fish meals per week. Aim for more, and include fatty fish for more omega-3 fat.
- Use organic free-range meats.
- Low-fat dairy products are a good source of protein and calcium.
- Include low-fat cheese in your afternoon snack.

FAT

Our bodies require fat for growth, manufacturing hormones, prostaglandins, cell membranes, immune responses, sexual development and reproduction, and mental health. We cannot live without fat in our diet but we need it to be the best.

Saturated fat comes from animal sources. Fat from fish is omega-3, which is an essential fat for all-around health. It protects the heart and mind by its anti-inflammatory actions. Plants contain fat in small amounts.

THE BENEFITS OF OMEGA-3, CALCIUM, AND PROTEIN

Essential to life and good health, omega-3 essential fatty acids protect against disease and can treat illness. Found in fish, omega-3 fats protect the heart and prevent inflammation in the body.

- Omega-3 fats increase levels of the good cholesterol, HDL, and lower the levels of bad LDL.
- Omega-3 fats reduce the risk of heart attack, arrhythmia, and sudden death.
- Omega-3 fats are anti-inflammatory.
- Omega-3 fats enhance skin elasticity and radiance.

> Keep your meals colorful with a variety of vegetables and fruit—you will be rewarded with renewed energy and health.

By eating a variety of fresh fruit and vegetables you will assure yourself of a steady supply of power molecules. You will be naturally full because the foods containing power molecules are high in fiber. The reason we have gotten away from eating this way is industrialization.

> Cans of tuna or salmon are economical and portable portein sources. Don't buy water-packed varieties that dilute the nutrients, or fish packed in soybean oil, which contains omega-6. Omega-3 and omega-6 fats compete for absorption in the body. Their molecular conformations are similar. If fish is packed with omega-6 oil, such as soybean oil, we are unable to absorb omega-3 fat completely. But omega-3 fat has a very different conformation than monounsaturated fat, so there is not competition between them for absorption. Look for fish packed in olive oil (monounsaturated fat) because it will allow you to absorb all the omega-3 fat present.

EXERCISE MAKES THE BIGGEST DIFFERENCE

Studies have shown that dieting can be effective in losing weight, but not nearly as effective or long-lasting as dieting in combination with exercise. Exercise helps to burn calories. If you're trying to lose weight, consider adding activities to your day to help accelerate the process.

SAMPLE ENERGY MENU

Breakfast
Two omega-3 eggs with 1½ ounces low-fat cheese and herbs, one slice whole grain bead with almond butter, fruit cup with colorful medley and mint. Coffee or tea.

Lunch
Soup of white beans and escarole. Organic chicken breast on salad of dark green leafy vegetables; red, yellow, and green peppers; and grated carrots. Add olive oil and vinegar to taste. Mineral water.

Afternoon snack
Handful of almonds with curry powder, one cup plain low-fat yogurt. Green tea.

Dinner
Grilled salmon with asparagus spears, brown rice with rosemary and orange segments. Side salad of sliced tomatoes, red onions, arugula, basil, and Italian balsamic vinegar. One glass red wine.

Dessert
Dr. Klauer's Omega-3 Cake (page 183) with raspberries.*

The cake described is my variation of the recipe by Ralph Holman, one of the early researchers in the benefits of omega-3 fat. It contains only the highest-quality ingredients when made in the manner I outline.

We have such bounty to choose from today. Explore the gourmet shops. You have to have variety in your diet. Be inventive and don't be afraid to try something new.

LOW-FAT, HIGH-ENERGY CHEESE SNACKS

- Organic Valley Stringles—Organic Valley produces 100 percent organic dairy products that are nutritious and good for you. Milk from pasture-raised organic cows has recently been shown to have significantly higher levels of vitamin E, omega-3 essential fatty acids, beta-carotene, and antioxidants than milk from conventional cows raised in confinement. Organic Valley Stringles are individually wrapped and available in Cheddar, Colby Jack, and mozzarella, and are perfect for a quick energy boost on the go. www.organicvalley.coop
- Cabot's Reduced Fat Cheddar—one-ounce serving has just seventy calories and 4.5g fat. www.shopcabot.com or www.cabotcheese.com for store locations.
- Calabro All Natural Fat Free Ricotta—Family-owned Connecticut cheese company makes 100 percent skim milk ricotta with no fat, salt, or preservatives. Try the fat-free mozzarella too. www.calabrocheese .com

GET THE SUGAR MONKEY OFF YOUR BACK!

Most people reading this will think, "I'm not addicted to sugar. I can stop eating sugar anytime I want." Living a sugar-free life may seem daunting at first. It is a real eye-opener for most people to actually realize how much sugar they have in a twenty-four-hour period. Very soon, many people revert back to their old ways and go rummaging through the snack cabinet looking for anything that can give them their sugar high. Most American consumers are so addicted to sugar that they will deny their addictions similar to the way a crack or heroin addict does. Sugar cravings may actually control their behavior.

TAKE MY SUGAR TEST

- What did you have for breakfast today? Sugar in your morning coffee? Pancakes or waffles with syrup? Sweetened cereal? Bran muffin? English muffin with jelly?
- What did lunch look like? Sweetened salad dressing from the salad bar? Pasta with tomato sauce? A slice of pizza? Hot dog with relish? Did you wash it down with a diet soda or flavored iced tea?
- What about dinnertime? A juicy burger with fries and ketchup? Barbecued chicken or ribs? Sweet-and-sour pork with a bowl of white rice? Did you have a cold beer or glass of white wine with your meal? A piece of apple pie à la mode for dessert?

It all adds up. Sugary snacks and foods create sugar junkies. When you have three meals a day loaded with sugar, you are seriously sabotaging your health. Sugar sneaks into a lot of foods you might not even imagine: Kellogg's All-Bran cereal has sugar as the second ingredient and high-fructose corn syrup as the third ingredient, Volvic water with orange essence contains sugar! Make it a point to read labels. Do you think that Fruit Roll-Ups are a healthy snack for your children? You won't after you read the label and find pear puree, corn syrup, and oil. It contains twelve carbohydrates, which are all sugar, or about three teaspoons of sugar in just one roll-up.

My energy plan eliminates processed food and unnecessary sugar. You may experience an initial period of adjustment where you intensely crave the toxic foods that were once part of your daily diet—just like an addict craving alcohol or other drugs of dependence. The reason is the excess sugar and drugs of abuse work in the same area of the brain, the hippocampus. Both cause cravings, initial euphoria, but later, a crash.

BREAKFAST REALLY *IS* THE MOST IMPORTANT
MEAL OF THE DAY

On most mornings, my high-profile patients are rushing out the door, either to a board meeting or to walk their dogs in the park, or to take their children to school. They don't always have time to sit down as a family and have a healthy breakfast.

A good breakfast that you can eat on the go can help set your energy level for the rest of your day. Your choice doesn't have to be either to skip breakfast, grab a coffee and croissant from the snack bar in your office building, or show up late for work. There are real energy benefits to eating a morning meal. A healthy breakfast may sharpen your mental abilities in the morning.

WHAT GOES INTO A "GET UP AND GO" BREAKFAST?

The first meal of the day should fuel your body until lunch. You should feel rested from a good night's sleep; now you need food that will revive and invigorate you. Aim for a long-lasting fuel source. The main things to look for in a healthy breakfast are protein and fiber. Those two things are key to feeling full and satisfied. Sugar gives you empty calories and nothing else. Sugar also causes a glucose/insulin surge with a crash about an hour later.

A healthy breakfast is one of the key behaviors for keeping your weight down. The National Weight Registry looked at people who had lost sixty pounds or more and kept it off for two years or longer and guess what? They all ate breakfast and they exercised. I suggest that you do both in the morning. A breakfast high in protein and fiber will keep you satisfied and working at your peak until lunch. Protein at breakfast suppresses gherlin, a hunger signal, more than carbohydrate. Gherlin is a hormone produced by the stomach in response to the sight of food, signaling hunger in the brain. Protein in the morning causes the gherlin level to fall and to stay suppressed for a longer time than carbohydrate.

HEALTHY ENERGY BREAKFAST

- Two omega-3 eggs with escarole and part-skim mozzarella omelet (25g protein, 1g fat, 150 calories)
- 1 slice whole grain toast with unsweetened jam
- ½ cup blueberries
- Skim latte

This breakfast will supply lasting energy all morning because it contains protein, which is digested more slowly than carbohydrate, and the carbohydrate that are present have fiber. Additionally, there are powerful omega-3s in the eggs and phytochemicals in the berries and escarole.

> Omega-3 fat can be found in the yolk of eggs when chickens are raised with flaxseed or other sources of omega-3 fat. Check the carton label and buy the omega-3 eggs.

CRASH 'N' BURN BREAKFAST

Contrast my healthy breakfast plan with the typical American fast food breakfast. For example: Dunkin' Donuts Egg and Cheese English Muffin Sandwich accompanied by Coffee Coolatta, which is actually one of the healthier choices on their menu. Let's analyze the breakfast using the principles I have outlined. The carbohydrate in the English muffin has no fiber. The cheese is American cheese, which has a good amount of protein but the quality of protein is not the best. But what I find shocking is that the "egg" in the sandwich is a mixture of whole egg, whole milk, soy oil, water, modified food starch, salt, xanthum gum, white pepper, and citric acid. You are not eating an egg but an egg batter! Dunkin' Donuts isn't the only place that uses this unusual mixture. In fact, most fast food restaurants use egg batter for their egg sandwiches. So if you thought that the taste was unusual, you now know why! The fast food interpretation of scrambled eggs is about as far as you can get from omega-3 eggs scrambled in a small amount of olive oil. What about the coffee? The Coolatta is a low-budget rendition of syrupy coffee drinks with sugar and calories you do not need. This breakfast offers little in the way of sustained energy. The breakfast described is high in calories, low in fiber, and substitutes artificial ingredients for real foods.

"I'M JUST NOT HUNGRY IN THE MORNING..."—I have heard that a million times. But you need to eat breakfast. Think of the word *breakfast*. You are break-ing the evening fast. The body has processed the food you gave it the day be-fore. Refuel your body with the best energizing foods.

Studies have shown that children who miss breakfast have trouble with reading, memory, and cognitive skills. In short, learning suffers when the brain is not receiving the fuel it needs.

THREE SQUARES AND A SNACK

Whatever you do, don't skip meals. Americans are eating fewer real meals but getting fatter. Instead of a structured mealtime, the trend is now to grab something and go. We have become grazers. If you graze you will gain. Un-like snacking, a quick pick-me-up between meals, grazing replaces meals. It is equivalent to eating throughout the day and, for many, it has replaced dining.

According to a recent study, during the workweek 17 percent of Ameri-cans will skip lunch, 13 percent will skip breakfast, and 6 percent will skip dinner.

IT'S NEVER TOO LATE

Exercise and healthy eating have benefits for all age groups. Look at what happened to Lillian. At seventy-three she was the senior vice pres-ident of a large marketing firm in New York City. She was referred by her friend because she wanted to lose about twenty pounds and feel less lethargic. Lillian lived alone in the suburbs. She had started work-ing when her husband passed away fifteen years before, as a way to keep busy. Now she was at the top of her field and wanted to get herself together. Lillian was intelligent, sharp as a tack, and even though her internist had failed to warn her about her steadily increasing weight, she knew it wasn't a good idea. And Lillian was right; at every age it is important to maintain your weight. Just because Lillian was in her seventies did not mean she had a green light to gain weight. Lillian ate the way many Americans eat; she consumed a high-carbohydrate diet with insufficient protein and calcium. She also did not exercise, something else her primary care physician had not advised her about. Lillian began the plan that I advise for many. She started her day with protein. Since she was rushing to work in the morning, she chose the all-natural yogurt and a piece of fruit for breakfast. Part of her job included taking important people to lunch. Every day she dined at Michael's, a literary hot spot on West Fifty-seventh Street. For lunch she had grilled fish or chicken and vegetables. Before commuting home, she would stop at the Peninsula spa for a workout. She used a trainer for weight training twice a week and the other days used the treadmill or elliptical machine for aerobic exercise. As Lillian saw how much better she could look and feel, she delighted in her new lifestyle. She truly became a woman on a mission. Because she was determined to spread the word, Lillian arranged for her firm to participate in a Central Park walk for lung cancer.

REFUELING YOUR BODY

The worst time of day for feeling fatigue for most people tends to be midafternoon. You had a good lunch at 12 P.M., and now it is 4 P.M. and you are dragging! Remember the four hours that it takes to digest a meal? Bingo. You are working on empty. Additionally, the hormones of the body are produced in a circadian rhythm. Normal secretion of insulin (a storage hormone) begins to rise in the afternoon. The rise in insulin causes you to feel hungry. That is why you will need a snack in the afternoon. But you can do a lot better than hitting the nearest vending machine, which is laden with empty-calorie snacks, candy, and chips that are sure to sabotage your energy supply. Turning to caffeine is not a good solution, either. Caffeine will give you a temporary jolt at best, which leaves you even more tired later on.

The trick is to choose a snack that will boost your energy level and keep it relatively constant for the rest of the afternoon. Eating processed sugar, found in sodas and candy, will give you a sugar spike and a quick charge. But a too-rapid rise in blood sugar can precipitate a sugar low, due to the large rush of insulin the body produces to deal with the sugar overload. The result is fatigue and hunger, likely leading you to overeat.

To keep yourself feeling energetic throughout the afternoon, choose something worthwhile. A handful of nuts is ideal. Include fruit, if you are still hungry. Another idea: a glass of skim milk or yogurt with a piece of fruit on the side. My afternoons tend to be very busy and my day starts early. Therefore, my solution to the energy slump in the afternoon is keeping Ziploc bags with walnuts and almonds (portion controlled, of course) in my desk. I find a cup or two of green tea enjoyable in the afternoon, and it gives me a lift. If you enjoy caffeine in the afternoon and it does not disturb your sleep, coffee is okay, too.

> When you get the munchies, try a handful of crunchy roasted pumpkin seeds rich in omega-3 to give you an instant energy boost.

HYDRATION, HYDRATION, HYDRATION!

Drinking sufficient water is essential for a healthy lifestyle. Physical and mental performance is directed by the body's state of hydration. I suggest drinking a minimum of two to three liters of water daily. When I say water, I mean water, pure H_2O. Mineral water is a good idea because it supplies extra calcium and the carbonation can be refreshing. It is surprising when someone asks, "You mean sparkling water counts as water?" Sure it does. In fact, mineral water has the added benefit of calcium. Perrier has 60mg calcium per liter, San Pellegrino 120mg calcium per liter, and San Faustino 400mg calcium per liter. Soda, coffee, and sugary drinks do not count.

WARNING SIGNS OF DEHYDRATION

- Fatigue
- Loss of appetite
- Flushing
- Light-headedness
- Burning in stomach
- Dry mouth
- Dry cough
- Heat intolerance
- Dark urine with strong odor
- Stumbling
- Shriveled skin
- Sunken eyes
- Muscle spasms
- Delirium

HOW MUCH WATER DO YOU NEED?

- Drink a minimum of two to three liters of water every day.
- Drink a large glass of water before exercise.
- Drink four to six ounces every fifteen to twenty minutes during exercise.

There is a debate in the medical community about how much water you really need daily. You get water from other things as well. If you are on a diet, you need more water to avoid kidney stones and bladder infections. I tell my patients to drink a lot because they are also exercising and need to stay hydrated.

When exercising you need to stay ahead of your fluid requirements. Drink a big glass of water before going to the gym. Just how much you should drink is debated by experts. The amount of perspiration is determined by genetics, sex, body size, medications, and how well you tolerate heat. Women perspire less than men. Keep a sports bottle with you during exercise and drink frequently from it every fifteen or twenty minutes. But just say no to sweet, sugary, or even diet drinks that contain artificial sweeteners.

WATER WITH A TWIST?

Hint Water is pure H_2O with a hint of natural flavors, including cucumber, peppermint, raspberry-lime, and pear. No sugar, no calories, no sodium, and refreshing flavor. www.drinkhint.com

---

WARNING

Read your labels, even when you buy water. Many flavored waters contain fructose and sugars to make them taste fruity.

Everyone is aware that they need to drink water during the summer. Do you know that you need even more water during the winter? The air cannot hold moisture when it is cold. When cold air is heated, the relative humidity can drop very low. Inside our offices and homes the humidity can bottom out. The problem with this situation is we then lose tremendous amounts of water just by breathing.

Our lungs naturally humidify oxygen that we breathe to approximately 100 percent humidity. Within our lungs we absorb oxygen in tiny air sacs, called alveoli. The thin-walled alveoli are only one or two cells thick. When we inhale dry air our body uses water to humidify it so that it comes close to 100 percent by the time it reaches the alveoli. When we exhale we give back some of the water as CO_2 exits the body, but not all of it. In normal humidity you can expect to lose one to two liters of water this way, but when the environment is dry, as it is in *every* heated building in the world, this can rise two- to fourfold. The net effect is that during the winter, indoors it is drier than the Mojave or Gobi deserts. When you exercise outdoors on a cold day the same process occurs. You breathe in cold air but the alveoli are just as sensitive to temperature as they are to humidity. So the body heats and humidifies the air before it reaches the alveoli. Don't forget that when you exercise you breathe faster, thus speeding up the dehydration process. Additionally, you lose body water through perspiration.

As you can see, the cold weather challenges our hydration daily. The idea is to stay in front of the fluid loss by drinking water throughout the day and avoiding alcohol.[1]

One of my patients, Rosa, goes to Spain every summer to visit her family. As you can imagine, July and August in Marbella get pretty hot and sticky. In order to stay hydrated, she freezes a case of twelve-ounce water bottles at a time (always leaving some room at the top of the bottle for expansion) and carries two with her when she is out and about in the Spanish sun. The water is frozen solid at first, but thaws quickly in the sun, and she always has a cold one to stay hydrated with and to cool her body down.

THE GREENING OF OUR DIET

Organic foods are now more in demand than ever before, prompting most grocery store chains to stock more natural foods. From pesticide-free produce to organic meat, there are many more options for the health conscious. But don't be fooled—there are no standardized definitions for the terms *all natural* or *natural*. The U.S.D.A. Web site has details on exactly what various organic labels mean.

Organic foods are produced according to certain production standards. For fruits and vegetables, it means they were grown without the use of synthetic pesticides, artificial fertilizers, human waste, or sewage sludge, and that they were processed without ionizing radiation or food additives. For animals, it means they were not the offspring of cloned animals. They were raised on 100 percent organic feed, were never given growth hormones or antibiotics, and their meat was never irradiated. Organic milk comes from animals that, for at least the past twelve months, were fed 100 percent organic feed and weren't given antibiotics or growth hormones. Organic eggs come from hens that were fed 100 percent organic feed and were never given growth hormones or antibiotics. Currently, the United States, the European Union, Japan, and many other countries require producers to obtain organic certification in order to market food as organic.

IT AIN'T NECESSARILY SO . . . ORGANIC

- **Organic seafood** doesn't mean a thing. The U.S.D.A. doesn't recognize the term.
- **Cage-free eggs** are from hens that are not confined to cages and possibly have access to the outdoors. It doesn't mean the eggs are organic.
- **Cage-free poultry** is a meaningless term because most chickens grown for meat are kept indoors cage-free until they are transported to slaughter.
- **Hormone-free** is an illegal term, since all animals naturally produce their own hormones.

PACKAGED FOODS

- One hundred percent organic. All the ingredients are organic.
- Organic. At least 95 percent of the ingredients are organic.
- Made with organic ingredients. At least 70 percent of the ingredients are organic.

Is organic produce better? The answer is complicated. The pesticides that kill insects have adverse effects on people who work with pesticides; farmers and those who work in fields have higher rates of asthma, Parkinson's disease, leukemia, lymphoma, and cancers of the stomach, skin, brain, and prostate.[2]

There are no studies of the risk to consumers from eating fruit and vegetables that contain presently used pesticide residues. The studies that exist document the risk from the older organochlorine pesticides, like DDT, chlordane, and heptachlor, which are stored in body fat. They remain in the body for years and increase the risk for non-Hodgkin's lymphoma and possibly prostate cancer.

While there are no present links of the current pesticides to the risk for disease, that doesn't mean that there are none. Just as some individuals are allergic to pollen and others are not, so it is with pesticides. Individuals have differing sensitivities to chemicals, and pesticides may trigger reactions in your body. Many people notice a difference in how they feel after switching to organically grown food. I don't believe anyone thinks pesticides are beneficial to us!

But more concerning is the effect the pesticides may have on children. Because children have smaller body volumes the pesticides become more concentrated. And because pesticides target the nervous systems of insects they may have an effect on the developing nervous system of children. Eliminate the "dirty dozen" of produce with the highest pesticide residues from your child's diet. Because children drink milk with their meals, it is important to make sure that it is organic.

As far as organic meat is concerned, the type of diet the animal has is just as important as whether the diet is organic. If steers are raised on organic grain it is an unnatural diet and will cause them to accumulate saturated and omega-6 fat within their bodies.

The Niman Ranch is a group of more than five hundred independent farmers who agree to raise their animals without antibiotics, hormones, and all of them graze freely in pastures. Prior to slaughter, the animals are fed grain for a short time. Niman Ranch produces consistently high-quality meat and is now being featured in high-end restaurants. Niman Ranch animals must be born in the United States. But, in the strict sense, it is not organic meat. www .nimanranch.com

From 2002 to 2004, the Washington-based nonprofit Environmental Working Group (EWG) analyzed the most commonly eaten fruit and vegetables and created a list of those with the highest pesticide levels. The list is a good guide for anyone who doesn't want to buy all organic, but who wants to avoid high-pesticide fruit and vegetables. This is especially important if you have small children.

TO BE AVOIDED

The Dirty Dozen

Peaches, apples, sweet bell peppers, celery, nectarines, strawberries, cherries, pears, grapes, spinach, lettuce, potatoes. The highest pesticide level was found in peaches. Because of the soft skin, pesticide residues were found within the flesh of the peach all the way through to the pulp.

The Cleaner Dozen
Lower-pesticide fruit and vegetables

Papaya, broccoli, cabbage, bananas, kiwis, sweet peas, asparagus, mangoes, pineapples, corn, avocados, and onions. Onions were pesticide-free!

To be certified organic, products must be grown and manufactured in a manner that adheres to standards set by the country they are sold in. In the United States, this means the National Organic Program (NOP) Standards. In the States, the Organic Food Production Act of 1990 (7 U.S.C.A. §6501–22) required that the U.S.D.A. develop national standards for organic products. The regulations (7 C.F.R. Part 205) are enforced by the U.S.D.A. through the National Organic Program under this act. These laws essentially require that any product that claims to be organic must have been manufactured and handled according to specific NOP requirements. A U.S.D.A. organic seal identifies products with at least 95 percent organic ingredients.

Organic products typically cost 10 to 40 percent more than similar conventionally produced products, but I assure you they are worth it. Farmers who grow organic food must meet stricter quality standards to have their products certified organic. More labor is required, which brings up the cost. I used to think organic didn't really matter, but I have come to believe that these are superior foods in terms of good health and nutrition.

CHAPTER FOUR

ENERGY BUSTERS: SUGAR, SUGAR, SUGAR!

TRANS FAT WILL KILL YOU

That's a simple fact. So you need to get educated about what you put in your body. Most people believe that they know everything about nutrition and just need a little help. The truth is that they usually don't know nearly as much as they think they do.

SIX STEPS TO DECIPHERING LABELS

To identify the energy boosters from the energy busters, let's take a closer look at how to read a label as a nutritionist does.

STEP ONE—SERVING SIZE

First look at the number of servings and the serving size because everything else you read will be based on the serving size. For example, the label lists two servings per container, but you may think it is only one serving and then proceed to eat the whole box. To avoid this, buy smaller packages or single-serving sizes whenever possible. If there is no readable label, look at the list of ingredients. Ingredients are listed in order of concentration, from high to low.

STEP TWO—CALORIES

Now look at the number of calories—per serving size.

STEP THREE—FAT

Pay attention to the total fat content on the label. As far as fat is concerned, limit the saturated kind. The bad unhealthy trans fats should also be listed. The difference between these and the total fat should equal up to the healthier mono- and polyunsaturated fats. These are the fats derived from fish or plant sources. Remember, the right fats in the right amounts are actually good for you. You want to keep saturated fat low—less than two grams of fat per serving.

Any trans fat should raise a red flag—don't buy it, don't eat it, and don't even consider bringing it home! If there is less than 0.5g trans fats, the manufacturer can list this as being zero, or trans-fat free. It can eventually add up. Unknowingly, you may be eating four or five snacks a day with 0.5g trans fats per serving—adding up to a few grams daily, something that can actually zap your energy reservoir and undermine your healthy eating plan.

JUST SAY NO TO TRANS FATS

Because of the bad reputation trans fats are receiving, some snack makers have responded by labeling their foods as "trans-fat free." Hopefully, the elimination of trans fats will make common financial sense to the manufacturer. It is simple Economics 101; if we didn't buy foods with trans fats and demanded healthier alternatives, manufacturers would have to figure out ways to make foods people would actually eat to keep their profits up.

STEP FOUR—CARBS

Now look at total carbohydrate. Zoom in immediately on *sugar*. Sugar content should be low. If you deduct the fiber and sugar from the total, you get the starch, which is basically sugar also. If twelve grams are listed as total carbohydrate and ten grams listed as sugar, then about 80 percent is simple sugar, which is not good. You want most carbs to be from *complex* carbohydrates, not from sugar, sweeteners, or syrups. Avoid high-fructose corn syrup and partially hydrogenated vegetable oil, and foods with a high-glycemic index in order to prevent sugar and insulin spikes. Many foods, like juices, are all natural yet very high in sugar. Be careful; it all adds up. Also locate the fiber content, which should be high. For example, in a cereal, look for more than four grams per serving.

STEP FIVE—PROTEIN

Now look at the amount of protein per serving. Protein is a building block of bones, muscles, cartilage, skin, and blood. For example, my Everyday Nutrition ready-to-drink shakes contain twenty grams protein, with high amounts of branched-chain amino acids (BCAA). BCAA are the most important amino acids in building and repairing muscle fiber. Studies have shown greater strength gains in athletes who consumed drinks with BCAA after working out.

PASTA PLUS

There are protein- and omega-enriched pasta noodles like Barilla Plus that have a healthier, lower glycemic index. Barilla Plus contains 10g protein, 4g fiber, and 180mg plant-based omega-3 fat. Their texture is somewhat different when prepared al dente. Lentil pasta is another innovation.

STEP SIX—CALCIUM

What about calcium? Calcium is essential for total body health. Calcium not only keeps your bones and teeth strong over your lifetime but also is essential for the heart, muscles, and nerves to function properly.

Calcium is listed as a percentage of the normal daily requirement. Up until age fifty the daily requirement of calcium is 1000 milligrams and the percentage is based on that amount. If the label says a product contains calcium 30 percent DV (Daily Value), the product contains 300 milligrams calcium. Learn to look for calcium on the labels.

Calcium is difficult to get into the body and requires vitamin D for absorption. In dairy products this is added. Actually, calcium in dairy products is easily absorbed, as opposed to calcium in supplemental form.

The next thing you must consider is ingredients. The ingredients will be listed in order of concentration. Watch out for sugar and its cousins, which I have already talked about. Those should be way down near the bottom of the label. And be on guard for the source of fat. The highest saturated fats are palm kernel oil, palm oil, and coconut oil. Hydrogenated and partially hydrogenated vegetable oils become trans fat. Remember, these are only listed if the amount is greater than 0.5mg.

That's all there is to reading the labels. Don't bother with the other confusing items, such as percentage of daily value. If you are eating in a healthy way, you will meet those daily value requirements and you will get your vitamins in a natural way. If you have a problem with salt raising your blood pressure, make sure the label doesn't have too much sodium. And do not add extra salt to your food.

BAD THINGS COME IN SMALL PACKAGES, TOO

Cookies and snacks now come in little packages that are touted to have only "100 CALORIES." Simply putting junk food into a smaller package does not make it a healthy food that you should eat! Smaller size just means fewer calories in the package; so basically it's just a smaller serving of the same chips, cookies, or pretzels. These snacks often contain high-fructose corn syrup as a sweetener, and are often loaded with sodium and saturated fat. What zaps your energy? Sugar!

100-CALORIE PACK OF OREO THIN CRISPS

Serving Size—1 package (23g)

Calories—100

Fat Calories—20

Total Fat—2g

Saturated Fat—0g

Trans Fat—0g

Polyunsaturated Fat—0g

Monounsaturated Fat—0g

Cholesterol—0g

Sodium—160mg

Total Carb—20g

Fiber—less than 1g

Sugars—9g

Protein—1g

BE YOUR OWN HEALTH ADVOCATE!

Bonnie's story was a sad one. She was referred to me by her psychiatrist. At forty-five, she was morbidly obese and suffered from depression. Her history began as a slim young woman in college when she became depressed. She was prescribed medications that caused her to gain weight. After college she married and became pregnant, continuing to take the medications. At age two, Bonnie's son was diagnosed with a rare cancer, causing blindness, and attends a special program. To hear Bonnie relate these facts made me want to help her even more. She was so brave to visit me in light of what challenges she faced on a daily basis. Thus far, Bonnie has exceeded all expectations. Although she took a multitude of medications that increase weight gain, she has managed to lose thirty pounds in three months. When we began I gave Bonnie a list of the foods that she should eat daily and those that she should avoid at all costs. After her first visit, she discarded three shopping bags of bad foods. One evening she did not have time to cook and went to Boston Market to pick up a grilled chicken for her family. As the clerk behind the counter packed up her order, he was about to include biscuits. Bonnie knew these were not going to help with her weight-loss plan, so she told the clerk that she did not want them. The clerk told her that they were included in the price and she had paid for them. She argued that if she had paid for them, then she would like to substitute a vegetable instead. The clerk told her that was not possible. Bonnie asked to speak to the manager but was told that he was unavailable. Bonnie left but as soon as she got home she e-mailed the headquarters with a complaint. Her complaint eloquently stated that since she was obese, she had requested broccoli as a substitute for the biscuits, and was refused. Bonnie later received an e-mail from the Boston Market headquarters with an apology and several gift certificates for meals. You must advocate for your own health, no matter what.

And, dear reader, if Bonnie did it, then so can you. Restaurants and food companies do not have your health as their priority, so it must become yours. If you do not take care of your health, who will?

LIQUID CALORIES

Did you know that drinking sugary drinks will actually make you thirstier?

Researchers at the Rudd Center for Food Policy and Obesity at Yale University found a clear association between soft drink intake and taking in more calories. The studies showed that, on days when people drink soft drinks, they consumed more calories than on the days when they did not have soft drinks.

Most of us don't compensate for the extra calories in sodas. For example, if you have a burger and a cola drink, you won't necessarily eat less of the burger—or fewer fries—than if you were washing the burger down with water. In some cases, people who regularly drink soft drinks eat even more. The additional calories they ingest may be more than the calories in their soft drinks. Sodas can lead to greater calorie intake because people grow accustomed to having a certain level of sweetness. That applies to diet sodas, too; they aren't any better because you are still stimulating the drive for sweetness. Drinking liquid calories is different from eating solid calories because they are not at all satisfying.

Drinking sugary beverages is not a healthy choice, and there are many better alternatives. Stimulation comes from artificial sources like caffeine, energy drinks, and sugar, which offer only a temporary, unsustainable high. This accounts for why a sugar binge is inevitably followed by a sharp decline in energy as you come down from the high.

BEST ENERGY BEVERAGES

It is a good idea to order sparkling water by the case, so you have it on hand. I order weekly cases of San Pellegrino from Fresh Direct, which delivers to my door. www.freshdirect.com

- Good old H_2O
- Green tea
- Ginger tea
- Sparkling mineral water with a lemon, a lime, or a splash of fruit juice

CAFFEINE—THE STARBUCKS GENERATION

If you think that we are drinking a great deal of coffee in the United States, you are right! The supermarket aisles are filled with an astonishing number of brands of coffee as well as newer coffee drinks. Traveling throughout the United States and even Europe, I was impressed by the numbers of people with an early morning Starbucks cup in their hands while hurrying to work. In my own neighborhood on the Upper East Side of Manhattan there are two Starbucks within three blocks of my apartment. And the coffee is consistently good!

The most widely grown coffee is coffee arabica. Most beans come from Central and South America, East Africa, and the Pacific. It might surprise you to know that coffee comes from the coffee berry. The bright red berries are picked, and then the bean must be separated and dried. The flavor of the coffee depends on the health of the plant and the soil. Because the arabica species is less hearty than the robusta species, its coffee taste is affected by drought and soil conditions. Coffee aficionados are able to distinguish origins and conditions just by taste!

During the roasting process the carbohydrate and fat within the bean are transformed into carbon dioxide and aromatic oils, unlocking the characteristic aroma and flavor.

Coffee can be purchased ground or as whole beans. I suggest that you purchase whole arabica beans, store them in the pantry (not the refrigerator) or freezer and grind them when you are ready to use them. The type of grind is dependent on how the coffee is to be brewed. If the brewing is very rapid, as in espresso machines, the coffee should be very finely ground. Drip and filter grinds are slightly coarser. And the French press uses the coarsest grind, as the coffee is in contact with the water for two to three minutes. The coffee percolator uses coarsely ground coffee as well.

Depending on the method of preparation, the caffeine content of a cup of coffee varies. The average amount of caffeine in a seven-ounce cup of coffee (with the exception of espresso) is given below:

- Drip coffee: 115 to 175mg
- Espresso: 100mg (serving size: one shot, 1.5 to 2 ounces)
- Brewed: 80 to 135mg
- Instant: 65 to 100mg
- Decaffeinated: 2 to 4mg

Most people drink caffeine because they enjoy the lift that it gives. Caffeine stimulates areas of the brain associated with alertness and causes release of epinephrine, a natural stimulant. We like to feel alert and vital. Caffeine also improves reaction time and athletic performance, as any athlete will attest. Many people who exercise early in the day make a point of drinking a cup of coffee, which is perfectly fine. Just drink a glass of water or two first to avoid fluid depletion.

Numerous studies have cited the health benefits of drinking coffee. The strongest benefit that I have seen comes from the reported association of coffee drinking with increased glucose sensitivity. Studies have suggested a protective effect against Parkinsonism. Evidence is increasing that higher coffee consumption may reduce the risk of type 2 diabetes.[1] Caffeine may reduce the risk of gallstones, colon polyps, and gout.

Caffeine has a long half-life of approximately nine hours. *Half-life* refers to the amount of time for half a drug to be metabolized. This means if you have a cup of coffee at noon, half the caffeine will remain in your system at 9 P.M. So if you are sensitive to the effects of caffeine it is best to limit your coffee intake to the mornings.

While on a book tour in Dallas for my first book, *How the Rich Get Thin,* I was scheduled as a guest for an early morning TV show. I stopped in a crowded Starbucks for my morning coffee. When my turn came the barista asked, "Good morning. What can I get you?" I answered, "I'll have a large skim latte, please." To which she responded, *not* "Would you like syrup?" but "What *kind* of syrup would you like?"! This was alarming to me. The barista assumed that syrup would go into my coffee. So many people turn a perfectly good drink like coffee or cappuccino or latte into a high-calorie, highly sweetened beverage. And when I observed the patrons, that was what they were all ordering, often topped with whipped cream. If you are going to drink coffee, keep it simple. Have a cup of coffee, an espresso, or a skim latte or cappuccino.

Coffee consumption can result in dependency and withdrawal symptoms. Those symptoms are headaches, difficulty concentrating, fatigue, lethargy, and irritability, proportional to the amount of coffee consumption; if you are a heavy coffee drinker they can include nausea and vomiting. There are times when it is necessary to stop drinking caffeine, however. A woman who is thinking of becoming pregnant should stop drinking coffee. If you are contemplating plastic surgery, your surgeon may recommend quitting coffee, as caffeine causes the capillaries to constrict, thereby reducing oxygen delivery to the healing skin. People with a history of heart arrhythmias or high blood pressure should not drink coffee. An overactive bladder will be stimulated by coffee and it should be avoided in those individuals.

If you are thinking of giving up drinking coffee I recommend the following two approaches:

- Dilute your coffee with decaffeinated coffee. Start with three-quarters regular beans mixed with one-quarter decaffeinated beans for three or four days, then half regular beans mixed with half decaffeinated beans for three or four days. Finally one-quarter regular beans and three-quarters decaffeinated beans. Keep in mind that decaffeinated coffee has a small amount of caffeine (approximately 5mg per cup); it should not be a problem but you might want to switch to herbal teas if zero caffeine is your goal. Within two weeks you will be caffeine-free!

- Or you can go cold turkey. Pick a three-day weekend and schedule activities that nurture you. Drink plenty of water, exercise, and have a massage. If your headaches are bothersome, take an aspirin. Avoid alcohol and empty calories to fill the caffeine void. Remember that chocolate contains caffeine, too, so it is not a suitable substitute. After three or four days you will be symptom-free.

HIDDEN CAFFEINE

TEA—Tea has lower amounts of caffeine than coffee. One eight-ounce cup of black tea contains 45mg versus the 110mg in a cup of black coffee. Green tea contains less—20mg of caffeine—and white tea is quite low at 15mg. Brewing tea longer than two minutes will increase the caffeine content. Instant tea drinks and bottled teas are a source of caffeine and lack the flavonoids and antioxidants naturally found in brewed tea.

Oddly enough, tea has actually become associated with a calming state of mind. Relaxing with a soothing cup of tea can be a welcome relief from the trials of the day. Tea contains the antioxidant and flavonoid catechin, and has been linked to a decrease in serious illnesses like heart disease and cancer. It also lowers cortisol, high levels of which can increase stress.

SODA—Bottled sodas have caffeine: a twelve-ounce can of Pepsi or Coke has about 35mg of caffeine. Mountain Dew, Josta, and Diet Coke have more. The popular energy drink Red Bull has as much caffeine as a cup of coffee.

CHOCOLATE—Chocolate contains caffeine in varying amounts. Example: Hershey's Special Dark Chocolate Bar: 1 bar—30mg.

ICE CREAM—If you are sensitive to caffeine, pay attention to what is in your frozen desserts:

- Ben & Jerry's Coffee Fudge No Fat Frozen Yogurt: 1 cup—85mg
- Starbucks Coffee Ice Cream: 1 cup—40 to 60mg
- Häagen-Dazs Coffee Ice Cream: ½ cups—58mg
- Starbucks Frappuccino Bar: 1 bar—15mg

MEDICINE—The medicine cabinet can also be stacked with caffeine-containing tablets. Some over-the-counter medications have significant amounts of caffeine.

- Excedrin: 2 tablets—130mg
- Anacin: 2 tablets—64mg

Prescription headache and migraine medications may also have caffeine, such as Fiorinal and Fioricet.

THE PERKS OF COFFEE

Coffee may even have some benefit to our health. Every morning I stop at a chic little neighborhood spot, Via Quadronno, for a skim latte. The Italian owners pride themselves on their coffee machine and would not dream of putting syrup in the espresso drinks. It reminds me of being in Rome!

In New York, coffee bars are everywhere. There is practically one on every block, and in some areas of the city, you can find three Starbucks within a two-block radius. Stronger coffee blends are actually taking on a new popularity. Organic coffee is also stirring up some interest.

3 CUPS FULL

The American Academy of Neurology has discovered that drinking three cups of coffee or tea a day can have a *protective* effect against memory decline in women age sixty-five and above (*Neurology*, August 7, 2007). They also found that the protection is even more dramatic as these women get older—from 30 percent lower likelihood of decline at sixty-five up to 70 percent above the age of eighty. Too bad it didn't have the same effect on men!

BEST COFFEE IN NEW YORK

- Via Quadronno—Italian coffee that brings you back to the *paninoteche* of Milan. 25 East Seventy-third Street. www.viaquadronno.com
- Jack Stirred Brewed Coffee—100 percent organic beans drip coffee to the stir brewer, a device created to oxygenate the grinds as they brew, supposedly reducing their acidity. 138 West Tenth Street
- McNulty's Tea and Coffee Co.—West Village landmark where full-bodied rich roasted beans are the norm. 109 Christopher Street. www.mcnultys .com
- Royal Coffee New York—Organic coffee importers offering specialty blends from Central America. 239 Western Ave., Staten Island. www.royalny.com

---

I enjoy drinking coffee but I don't rely on coffee for my energy. I get my energy from eating healthy fresh food, doing daily exercise, and making sure I get enough sleep. Coffee enhances what I am already doing. That is the point: Many people rely on coffee *exclusively* for their energy. Their energy levels are low because they have not fueled themselves with what the body requires. They are dragged down by a high-sugar and high-fat American diet and by a sedentary lifestyle. Because they have so little natural energy they require caffeine to function. The reason coffee- and caffeine-filled drinks are so popular is we have drained our energy reserves with inadequate sleep, poor food, and insufficient exercise. Turn this around and you will feel naturally energetic on a permanent basis. I witness this transformation in my patients daily.

BEWARE FLAVORED COFFEE DRINKS

Hot and iced coffee drinks may be flavored with sugary syrups such as chocolate, almond, hazelnut, cinnamon, and vanilla. Avoid these— they just add sugar!

COFFEE LINGO—GET TO KNOW YOUR
CUP OF JOE

- *Café au Lait*—A shot or two of espresso with steamed milk. Since you don't know if the milk is organic or loaded with fat, ask for low-fat or skim milk and inquire if the milk is organic.
- *Caffè Americano*—A shot of espresso diluted with hot water.
- *Caffè Latte*—A shot of espresso with steamed milk and lightly topped with foamed milk, so you could be getting a lot of fat if you're not careful. My favorite morning beverage is a skim latte.
- *Caffè Mocha*—A shot of espresso with chocolate syrup, steamed milk, topped with foamed milk or whipped cream.
- *Cappuccino*—A shot of espresso with steamed and foamed milk. My drink of choice after dinner is a decaffeinated skim cappuccino.
- *Espresso*—A concentrated coffee beverage produced with a method of brewing that uses pressure, rather than gravity, to pass hot water through a special blend and roast of ground coffee beans. Espresso is usually measured in "shots" of about 1 to 1½ ounces.
- *Espresso Macchiato*—A shot of espresso topped with foamed milk to keep it warm.
- *Espresso con Panna*—A shot of espresso topped with whipped cream.
- *Lungo*—Espresso that has been "run long," so more water is passed through the grinds. It is milder than a regular espresso and comes in a slightly larger portion.
- *Ristretto*—A "short run" of espresso, meaning a smaller, slightly stronger shot.
- *Schizo Coffee*—A cup of coffee that includes equal parts of decaffeinated and regular coffee, ideal if you are trying to cut down your caffeine intake.

THE PITFALLS OF SO-CALLED ENERGY BARS
AND DRINKS

Energy bars and protein bars were originally designed for athletes and outdoor enthusiasts who need snacks on the run. The problem that I have with them is that they are often little more than empty calorie snacks masquerading as energy enhancers. Some of these bars are intended to replace meals entirely. But they can be packed with sugar, artificial ingredients, and calories, so be conscious of what you are putting in your mouth. I suggest choosing a bar with natural ingredients such as nuts, honey, dates, cocoa, etc. The standard variety is about two hundred calories but that increases depending on the type of bar you choose. Watch the fat, keep it below 5g; avoid bars containing any trans fat and saturated fat.

HEALTHY BARS

These are some healthier, energizing alternatives:

- *Lärabar*—Organic, unsweetened fruit, nuts, and spices, one serving of fruit, with no added sugar, unprocessed, gluten-free, dairy-free, soy-free. One bar is 1.8 ounces, two hundred calories. Comes in yummy flavors like key lime pie and cherry pie. www.larabar.com
- *Gnu Bar*—Made with organic whole wheat flour, great as a cure for constipation, high in fiber. One Gnu Bar gives you 12g soluble and insoluble fiber. Low fat with only 130 to 140 calories per bar. www.gnufoods.com
- *Clif Bar*—Made with 70 percent healthy, organic ingredients, such as rolled oats, roasted soybeans, milled flaxseed, and soy flour, a mix of carbs, protein, and fiber and a moderate glycemic index. www.clifbar.com
- *Luna Bar*—From the makers of Clif Bar, this range of organic products is marketed for women; also comes in a whole grain morning nutrition bar for breakfast on the go. www.lunabar.com
- *Everyday Nutrition Bar*—My own recipe made from omega-3 nuts, whole grains, high in protein, and has a good amount of plant-

based omega-3 fat, so it gives sustained energy. www.janaklauermd
.com

ENERGY DRINKS

Energy drinks are, in theory, designed to give you a burst of energy by
using a combination of methylxanthines (including caffeine), B vitamins, and
exotic herbal ingredients. Energy drinks commonly include caffeine, guarana
(extracts from the guarana plant), taurine, various forms of ginseng, maltodex-
trin, inositol, carnitine, creatine, glucuronolactone, and ginkgo biloba. Some
contain high levels of sugar, although many brands also offer an artificially
sweetened version. These drinks are typically marketed to young people, and
people "on the go." Approximately 65 percent of energy-drink users are under
the age of thirty-five, with males representing approximately 65 percent of the
market. Many of the energy drinks available today have very high sodium levels as well.

BUZZ BEVERAGES

According to *Consumer Reports*, the average amount of caffeine found
in an energy drink is about 80mg per 8 ounces, as compared to
100mg in a standard cup of coffee.

MY PRIDE AND JOY—EVERYDAY
NUTRITION SHAKES

I've built my medical practice on the science of successful healthy eating
and teaching my patients about the rewards gained from a lifetime commitment to health, fitness, and nutrition. When I began my nutritional practice I
was surprised to find that the meal replacements available to physicians contained sugar as the second ingredient and high-fructose corn syrup. It was an
uphill battle. So, I decided to develop my own. My goal was to create a product
that was enriched with omega-3 fat, calcium, and protein and contained the

highest-quality ingredients. Everyday Nutrition shake is a ready-to-drink omega-3, protein, and calcium-rich meal replacement.

Everyday Nutrition shakes are the culmination of years of research. They are portable, they taste delicious, and they provide essential nutrients that your body needs to get going in the A.M. If you are now at your goal weight, these shakes make a great breakfast and a healthful snack or lunch on the go.

Everyday Nutrition shakes help your body to be strong and slim by supplying the nutrition that is often neglected.

- Omega-3 fat protects your heart and fights inflammation in the body. Everyday Nutrition is the *ONLY* ready-to-drink meal replacement with omega-3.
- Calcium is essential for total body health. Calcium not only keeps your bones and teeth strong over your lifetime but also is essential for the heart, muscles, and nerves to function properly. Calcium helps with weight loss and targets abdominal fat.
- Protein is a building block of bones, muscles, cartilage, skin, and blood. Everyday Nutrition shakes contain 20g protein, with high amounts of branched-chain amino acids (BCAA). BCAA are the most important amino acids in building and repairing muscle fiber.

WATCH OUT FOR MSG

Tara was a fifteen-year-old young lady attending an exclusive school on Manhattan's East Side who was accompanied by her mother to my office. Tara was not doing well in school and was exhausted by the end of the day. Tara appeared shy and slightly apprehensive. Her blood work showed no evidence of illness. Her physical examination was also normal for a fifteen-year-old female. But I had the feeling that something was a little off. Tara told me that her energy was very low. She dragged herself out of bed at 7 A.M. and struggled at school to stay awake. She told me of her love of biology and that she had won the science prize at school two years in a row. It disturbed her to feel herself so unmotivated and she was falling behind in her work. Tara experienced headaches several times per week. Tara's family customarily visited Mr. Chow's, a New York landmark Chinese restaurant, on Sunday evenings. They loved the excitement of the noodle preparation. For those who don't know, the Sunday evening noodle show is signaled by a gong at eight followed by the chef preparing noodle dough through elaborate tosses several feet into the air. It really is quite a show! Recently, Tara noticed that her asthma symptoms were worsening, especially on Sunday nights, after she visited Mr. Chow's.

I suspected that MSG was the root of her Sunday evening distress. Indeed, that proved to be the case. Tara's sensitivity to MSG caused her to have trouble breathing, requiring her to use her inhaler. But the medication in the inhaler prevented her from falling asleep. Tara was exhausted from a poor night's sleep; she was tired and had a headache the next day, which was Monday. Sleep-deprived, she could not do her best in school, which triggered stress hormones in her body. In an attempt to keep herself alert, Tara had begun drinking diet sodas containing caffeine, which made the problem worse because caffeine interfered with her sleep. By Friday, she was in serious sleep debt. It was a vicious cycle. Tara was doing poorly at school all because of a chemical in food!

I emphasized the importance of avoiding the MSG to Tara and her mother. They were surprised to learn that the chemicals in diet soda were MSG cousins. Glutamate can also cause a reaction in someone who is sensitive.

MSG is recognized as safe by the FDA and the American Medical Association for most people. But if someone has sensitivity, as Tara does, all forms of glutamate should be avoided. I taught Tara to read labels and to look out for MSG and its cousins. The FDA now requires that foods containing MSG state this on the label.

Other sources of free glutamates (MSG cousins) that can trigger sensitivity reactions in those people who have trouble with MSG are:

- Yeast extract
- Autolyzed yeast
- Hydrolyzed protein
- Aspartame

WHAT IS MSG?

MSG was first produced by a Japanese company as a flavor enhancer. It has been proposed that it represents a new taste, *umami*, or savory. This is felt to be distinct from all other tastes. MSG is made by fermenting starch, corn, sugar beets, molasses, or cane sugar to free the naturally occurring glutamate, then creating sodium salts of glutamate. MSG is a natural derivative with individuals exhibiting a range of sensitivities to it.

MSG has been in use in the United States since the 1950s, having been introduced as the kitchen seasoning Accent. It now is used in Chinese restaurants. Because it is a flavor enhancer, MSG can improve the taste of poor-quality meats. This has led to the use of MSG in a wide variety of fast food restaurants.

Beware: If you are sensitive to MSG, you can have severe headaches, flushing of the skin, nausea, rapid heart rate, and difficulty breathing.

CHAPTER FIVE

EVERYDAY ENERGY PLAN

A goal without a plan is just a wish.
—ANTOINE DE SAINT-EXUPÉRY

The first two weeks of the plan involve eliminating from your life all the factors that contribute to a fatigue state. By eliminating the fatigue factors the metabolism resumes a naturally energetic state. Poor sleep, excess alcohol, processed foods, and inactivity must be eliminated. And make no mistake about it, you will miss them! It is similar to a detox regimen because initially you will crave the foods and behaviors that you have become accustomed to. But as your body begins to adjust to the new food and behaviors, you can expect to feel better with renewed energy. In fact, you will feel better than you have in years! So what are you waiting for? Let's get going!

STEP ONE—SPRING CLEANING

The idea is to set up an environment that will support your new way of life, not sabotage it. Let's start in the kitchen. You want to be surrounded by only the best. Clean out your cupboard and refrigerator. Throw away all the energy-draining foods that are filled with preservatives, sugar, corn syrup, and bad fats. Toss the chips, sugary cereals, candy, cakes, crackers, snack foods, and anything that has high-fructose corn syrup or partially hydrogenated vegetable oil into the garbage can. Get rid of cake mixes, instant coffee, instant iced tea, and all sodas (including diet soda), noodles, spaghetti, white rice, and white bread and rolls. Discard any corn oil, vegetable oil, and ready-made salad dressings. Clean the shelves and put down fresh shelf paper.

FRIDGE FREEDOM

The refrigerator is next on your hit list.

Start with the freezer. Throw away ice cream, frozen yogurt, popsicles, frozen desserts, pie shells, frozen cookie dough, frozen TV dinners (even if they are diet dinners), old frozen leftovers, and frozen fish sticks.

In the refrigerator, throw away cream, full-fat milk, fat-free half-and-half, sweetened yogurts (even if they are "low calorie" or light yogurts), butter, margarine, artificial whipped topping, bologna, processed meats, American cheese, salad dressings, mayonnaise, any leftovers, and old food.

> What could be bad about fat-free half-and-half? If you look at the ingredients, to your surprise, you will find that it is made from skim milk, corn syrup, and a long list of artificial ingredients that give it the consistency of the high-fat variety. Fake ingredients and corn syrup make fat-free half-and-half a poor choice. You want only the best—natural, healthy foods!

Thoroughly wash the refrigerator and freezer using biodegradable soap. Replace all lightbulbs with energy-efficient varieties. You will be doing our environment a favor and you will be surprised at the amount of money that you will save on your electric bill.

BUILD A BEDROOM SANCTUARY

For your bedroom, serene should be the mood you are going for. The bedroom is to be your oasis of calm and rest. If there is a television in your bedroom, please have it removed or vow to watch only in the morning. If noise is a problem, invest in a white noise machine, which sounds like the steady hum of a fan on a slow speed. Alternatively, try a sound machine with the soothing sounds of nature: summer night sounds, gentle rainstorm, or ocean waves.

The best environment for sleep is darkness. Darkness stimulates the pineal gland to release melatonin, the hormone that induces sleep. Consider blackout shades if the streetlights shine into your bedroom. In the morning, you want to naturally awaken in response to light. An alarm clock is jarringly unpleasant. If you cannot wake up without an alarm, try a light alarm. You can program the device so that your bedroom gradually becomes lighter, over ten minutes to two hours' time. A light alarm simulates the effect of the sun's light, which awakened the world long before alarm clocks were invented. The Bio-brite Digital SunRise Alarm Clock will gently awaken you with a simulated sunrise. www.biobrite.com

When you are able to sleep late, or when you are on vacation, close your blinds completely to avoid any light peeking through to wake you. You can also wear a soft silky sleep mask infused with lavender for extra calm. Some of my patients who have young children, pets, or live in a hectic, noisy household, even use earplugs in desperation when they need to get their rest.

Is your mattress more than ten years old? If so, consider purchasing a new mattress. The mattress should give you firm support and it should be long enough for your height. Most couples are more comfortable in a king-size bed (which is actually the size of two twin beds) than in a queen size. This is especially true if your husband or partner is over six feet tall. A full-size bed for more than one adult is usually too cramped and doesn't leave enough room to stretch out.

Nothing feels better than flopping into a warm cozy bed and getting a great night's sleep. In European hotels, a feather bed is de rigueur. As the term suggests, feather beds are made from down feathers. It is placed on top of the mattress, and then the bottom sheet is placed over the feather bed and tucked under the mattress. A traditional feather bed is about four inches thick and stitched in channels or a baffle box design. With this much cushioning, even a rock hard mattress can feel soft and cuddly. It envelopes you in the most luxurious environment possible for sleep. You should shake out a feather bed weekly and turn it over to keep the fill evenly distributed.

Pure cotton bed linens with a high thread count of three hundred or above will last you a lifetime. Thread count is the number of threads per square inch. Hold the sheet up to the light and if you can see through the fabric, it is a sign that the thread count is on the low side. Generally, the higher the thread count, the softer and silkier the fabric feels. It is also more durable and washes better without losing its softness. Learn to care for them as they should be washed and ironed weekly. When ironing, use lavender water to give a calming scent.

Avoid electric blankets as they are suspected of disrupting energy flow. Wrap yourself in a fluffy down comforter or wool blankets for warmth.

Keep your bedside table free of clutter. On my own bedside table, I have a lamp, a telephone, and a picture of my family. The photograph is the last thing I see before turning off the light and the first thing that I see in the morning.

Always open a window in the bedroom, even if for just a few moments. We need fresh air in our bedrooms. Always have fresh flowers in soothing colors or a plant in the bedroom.

GO DON'T GO TO BED ANGRY

One common phenomenon I see among my patients is that they fiddle around on their computers too late in the day, start a project in which they get engrossed, and can't put the computer away to go to bed at a reasonable hour. By the same token, avoid having arguments with your partner or children in the evening, or you will toss and turn all night thinking about it. Make a rule to avoid any anxiety-provoking discussions after 6 P.M.

GET ORGANIZED

Put an end to disorganization in your closets and follow the rule, "If you haven't worn it in the last year, you don't need it." Organize the closets by color with the darker colors at one end graduating through the spectrum to the lighter colors at the other end. Seeing your clothes arranged in an organized fashion is pleasant and will save time in the morning. You want to be able to instantly locate what you will wear.

Your closet needs to be edited down. Then it should be categorized: shirts should be hung, short-sleeved, then long-sleeved, skirts, and pants. Follow the color palette of light to dark. I really think most people need to visit a closet store like The Container Store. Organization is very important. Use clear Lucite boxes for shoes. Or if you are using shoe boxes, have photographs on the outside of the shoe box. Polish all your shoes.

Use dividers at the top of the closet to keep folded shirts in line, and sweaters neatly stacked. Use a template to fold them so they are all the same size. The finer stores do this so all looks harmonious. Hang potpourri balls or cedar in the closet to give a lovely scent. You can easily make your own with oranges and cloves—which is a great rainy day project for kids.

Take clothes out of dry cleaner bags—the chemicals are harmful to fabrics when kept in an enclosed area. Fabrics need to breathe. Return the bags and hangers to the cleaners; it's good for the environment. Use only wooden or cedar hangers, *and* avoid wire hangers, as we learned from Joan Crawford. Clothes from the previous season should be stored in cloth bags after being inspected for dirt or makeup.

BATHROOM BREAKDOWN

Clean your medicine cabinet of old medications that have expired. Throw away any sleeping pills—you won't need those anymore if you follow my plan.

Your bathroom should have a full-length mirror so that you are able to assess your body unclothed. This idea is taken from the renowned designer, Bill Blass, and it makes perfect sense. Every bathroom in Bill Blass's homes featured a full-length mirror because he deemed it essential.

Relaxing baths and pampering are a treat and you deserve it. Add lavender bath salts to a warm bath and soak your anxiety away. Keep aromatic candles in the bathroom.

Your bathroom medicine cabinet should always have floss for your teeth. Floss at least once per day. Glide is the best product I have found; it doesn't shred or get stuck.

WORKOUT WISDOM

Join a gym. It is critical to line this up. No more excuses. Get yourself a good pair of sneakers and a pedometer. You are going to be an active person with energy. Consider enlisting a friend as a walking partner. Whatever works best for you, schedule it into your energy program. (Read chapter 8, "The Energy Workout.")

The bottom line—if you want to have more energy, you must exercise every day of your life. Period.

STEP TWO—GO SHOPPING

Make your grocery list of energizing foods. Bring this with you to the store, and tick off each item as you go!

- Fruit—Apples, apricots, berries (all kinds), melons (not watermelons), kiwis, figs, limes, oranges, lemons, peaches, pears, pomegranates, star fruit. Avoid bananas and grapes just for now. Bananas and grapes are high on the glycemic index, causing spikes in blood sugar. The most important fruits are berries. Be sure to eat berries every day.
- Vegetables—Artichokes, arugula, and asparagus (use thick asparagus spears for broiling or sautéing; use thin asparagus spears for steaming), green beans, peppers, bok choy, broccoli, Brussels sprouts, carrots, cauliflower, celery, collard greens, cucumbers, endive, eggplants, escarole, fennel, jicama, kale, kohlrabi, leeks, lettuces—the darker the better and never iceberg—mushrooms, onions, radicchio, radishes, seaweed, snow peas, spinach, sprouts, squash, sweet potatoes, Swiss chard, tomatoes, watercress. The most important vegetables are leafy greens—be sure to eat some daily.

- Herbs—Get creative. I use all kinds: chives, cilantro, parsley, rosemary, thyme, etc.
- Nuts—Almonds, Brazil nuts, cashews, pistachios, and walnuts.
- Condiments—Invest in good-quality extra-virgin olive oil. The bottle should be small and show a harvest date. Many people buy olive oil in large bottles to avoid running out of it, without realizing that olive oil begins to become stale after one year. Purchase a few high-quality vinegars for making salad dressings. Walnut oil, almond oil, and flaxseed oil are healthful also. One of my favorite oils is grapeseed oil. Grapeseed oil has a high smoking point so it cooks well.

> Low-fat salad dressing that comes in a spray bottle may sound like a great idea, but buyers beware. For example, Wish-Bone Salad Spritzers come in seven flavors. The Balsamic Breeze sounds harmless enough at one little calorie per spritz, but high-fructose corn syrup is the third ingredient listed! So if you are keen to take advantage of the portion-control aspects of this novel dressing device, just make your own. Williams Sonoma has an oil mister ($15 at www.williamssonoma.com) designed for spraying foods with a fine mist of oil with a built-in filter for herbs and garlic. Just fill your mister with your own favorite oil and toss in some finely chopped parsley or other fresh herbs and some garlic, and you're good to go. See my recipe for Great Grapes Dressing on page 186.

- Beverages and Water—Water is essential for health. Have the quality of your drinking water evaluated. If you live in a home with well water, it is important to have it checked as contamination from bacteria is a concern. If you live in the suburbs, I suggest that you call your local water department to find out about the quality of your drinking water. In an urban area, water is more likely from a metropolitan water system supplying thousands of homes. In New York City we are fortunate to have superb, highly palatable water. But in old New York apartment buildings the water pipes can result in brownish tap water. A good solution is a water filtration system, such as reverse osmosis.

- For bottled water choose mineral water that is bottled at the source. I am fond of San Pellegrino sparkling mineral water from Italy. Whether from the tap or bottled, make water your new drink of choice.
- Buy fresh coffee beans and grind them yourself at home for added freshness. Also get an assortment of green and black teas, and decaffeinated herbal teas.
- Grains—During Phase One, consume only the following grains: Brown rice, wild rice, quinoa, amaranth, whole wheat, spelt, wheat germ, and rye. Include products made from these grains only, such as bread, cereals, crackers, tortillas, wraps, and pasta.
- Dairy aisle—Stick with organic varieties only. Buy skim or 1 percent milk, low-fat cheese, low-fat or fat-free cottage cheese, and fat-free yogurt (free of sweeteners). Parmigiano-Reggiano makes a delicious snack and topping for salads; true, it is not fat-free but the flavor is intense, resulting in less chance of overconsumption.
- Canned and packaged foods—Buy pop-top four-ounce cans or packages of tuna and salmon, sardines, and chicken broth. Purchase fish that is packed in olive oil as opposed to water or vegetable oil. Water will leech away the omega-3 fat, and vegetable oil, an omega-6 fat, competes for absorption with omega-3. You want to take every opportunity to get the healthy omega-3s into your diet!

Parmigiano-Reggiano is a hard cheese made from cow's milk that is cooked but not pressed and comes in a big wheel. It originates from Parma and Reggio Emilia, Italy. Traditionally, the cows have to be fed only on grass or hay, producing grass-fed milk. It has a rich, fruity, and almost nutty flavor and a slightly gritty texture, which makes it delicious when grated over pasta, stirred into soup, eaten in chunks with balsamic vinegar, or shaved over vegetables and salads. This is not the same product as the grated Parmesan cheese found in typical supermarket varieties that comes in a cardboard can with a sprinkle top. These are usually aged for a short period, often contain extra sodium and added starch, and are sold grated so they lose their freshness quickly.

EATING GREEN

If you want to stay healthy, you need to have a lot of plants in your diet. My Energy Eating Plan can be adopted by vegetarians. Most important, you need adequate protein and you must find a source for the omega-3 fats. If you don't eat red meat, you need to eat fish daily. If you don't eat fish, then you must rely on omega-3 eggs for DHA. If you don't eat fish or eggs, you can get omega-3 short-chain fats from green plants, for example, kale or Swiss chard, and from walnuts.

WHAT IS A VEGETARIAN?

Quite simply, a vegetarian follows a plant-based diet. The most famous vegetarian of all time was Benjamin Franklin, though support for the vegetarian movement expanded considerably in the nineteenth century and by the twentieth century had reached widespread acceptance.

The term vegetarian encompasses a wide spectrum of eating habits. Basically, the universally eaten foods are: grains, vegetables, legumes, fruits, and seeds, with varying amounts of dairy products, with or without eggs.

There are two types of vegetarianism: lacto-ovo- and lacto-vegetarians. Lacto-ovo-vegetarians eat dairy products and eggs. Lacto-vegetarians do not eat eggs but eat dairy products and plant-based food only. Both types of vegetarians avoid meat, poultry, fish, and seafood. Pesco-ovo-lacto-vegetarians eat the meat of fish in addition to dairy products and eggs.

WHAT IS A VEGAN?

Vegans do not use any animal products. Some vegans do not use honey.

WHAT IS A PESCATARIAN?

Pescatarians, or pesco-ovo-lacto-vegetarian, is the names for fish-eating vegetarians. Fish is a great source of protein and contains omega-3 fatty acids, which may help lower your risk for heart disease. Unlike red meat, all fish are very low in saturated fat. Some white-meat fish (sole, haddock, cod, and flounder) are also very low in calories and fat.

STEP THREE—EVERYDAY ENERGY JOURNAL

When I see someone in my Park Avenue office I give them a journal. I ask them to record their goal for the day, when they wake up and go to bed, what food they consume and at what time, and the type and duration of their exercise. This accomplishes two things:

1.   A journal is an accounting, of sorts. If you eat it, you write it down. The journal chronicles sleep and exercise. It causes you to become superaware of what you do. Your goals and activities are in black and white. Up until this point, I have driven the plan—but with the journal you record what you have chosen. Is it healthy and energy promoting or not? The journal is the record.

2.   A journal keeps you on the four-hour plan, which may seem unnatural until you establish the rhythm. Eating good food at regular four-hour intervals will keep your energy elevated. When you write your goal for the day, you articulate your aspirations and give them power.

See Appendix on page 207 for the Everyday Energy Journal.

EVERYDAY ENERGY NUTRITION JOURNAL

Date

Your Goal for the Day: Take a moment to think about what you want to accomplish today and write it down. Writing down your goal signifies your commitment.

Awakening: Record the time you woke.

Exercise: Record activity and duration.

Breakfast: Record time and what you ate.

Lunch: Record time and what you ate.

Afternoon Snack: Record time and what you ate.

Dinner: Record time and what you ate.

Alcohol Intake: Record every drop!

Glasses of Water: Record (ten glasses).

Bedtime: Record the time you went to bed.

The journal is a very important tool. The journal is a record of your commitment. Don't skip this! Whatever you write down is real, and this has worked brilliantly for my patients.

You can log on to www.janaklauermd.com to find a journal template that may be downloaded and printed or kept on your computer. A scaled-down version of it is printed in the back of this book. Of course, you can just write everything down in a beautiful notebook if you prefer. Some of my patients carry it with them in their handbags. Do follow the guide given above as all of the components—sleep, exercise, foods, and the times you ate—are important for optimal functioning.

Keep your journal with you and enter the foods right after eating them. It really is more accurate than just relying on your memory. Don't worry about portion sizes right now. Instead, focus on eating the recommended foods. Be sure to record your exercise activity and duration. Don't worry if you are doing "enough" or "the right kind" of exercise. At the beginning of the plan your goal should be to establish a pattern of prioritizing daily exercise. For now, just be consistent and once you have your pattern established, you will naturally want to increase the duration and intensity. In fact, by committing to daily exercise you will be doing more than 90 percent of the American population.

Step Four—Prioritizing

Many of us are overachievers, but even if your to do list is a mile long, you can always find room to pare down to what needs to be done immediately. Set priorities that match your current energy level, and cut out anything on your list that depletes your precious energy supply!

- When your energy is low, take a hard look at your list and prioritize. Decide what can wait until tomorrow and what is really urgent to do at that moment.
- Take advantage of an unexpected energy spurt to get on a roll and finish those nagging little tasks that you have been putting off for ages.
- Assess all your obligations and determine which are really important and meaningful for you, and which are nice to do but nonessential. A false sense of obligation or guilt can make you say yes to invitations or tasks

that you would rather avoid. Spending quality time with a close friend can give you a feel-good boost, but having to attend a distant acquaintance's husband's funeral might drag you down when you are already dragging. Find time to do the things that bring you enjoyment and satisfaction.

- Identify the times of day when you are most productive. Are you a morning person? Or do you come alive after dark? Try to work with your natural inclination and internal time clock whenever possible, instead of fighting it. For example, if you can't function well before 9 A.M., schedule important meetings for mid-morning.

- Learn to be your own time-management coach. Plan your days, weeks, and months in advance, and determine where you can afford to cut back if needed. Add some extra family time into your weekly schedule; your kids will definitely appreciate it.

- Unexpected events such as a financial setback or the loss of a loved one can cause plenty of stress and drain you of much-needed energy. This is a good time to seek counseling to help you heal, and get you back on track toward feeling stronger emotionally and otherwise. Emotional health goes a long way toward improving your outlook on life and your resultant energy levels.

- Don't be afraid to say no to projects that you simply don't have time for. While this may not always be possible at work, a supervisor or colleague often appreciates honesty up front, rather than finding out a task has gone unfinished right before an important deadline.

- Give yourself a cushion. There will always be unexpected crises or changes in plans, so be careful not to pack your schedule so tight that any small setback will cause chaos. Schedules that are booked every hour on the hour are an obvious setup for your ultimate energy depletion.

- Ask for help if you need it. You simply can't do everything by yourself, nor should you be expected to. Sometimes you can be your own worst enemy by putting undo pressures on yourself to constantly achieve more. Give yourself a break.

Make sure you maintain consistency in these three key areas of your routine: diet, exercise, and sleep. You will perform the tasks on your list with more energy and feel more prepared to take on life's daily challenges.

PHASE ONE—BEGIN YOUR ENERGY PLAN

It's showtime! Let's assess the journey you have undertaken.

First, you made the decision to change your life. You thought it through and decided to take action. You want a more energetic life; in fact, you are tired of being tired. Others may have just wished that they could change things, but you decided that you would take action. You know it will be rough but the hardest part is just getting started, shifting the way you live each day into a pattern that will nurture your health and give you the energy that you are meant to feel.

Second, you have structured your environment to ensure success. This is very important because it means you have eliminated foods and clutter that were toxic to health. Your journal will record your progress. You have structured your environment around self-love and reverence for health. You have made the decision to care for the vessel of your spirit, your body. Now you can put the plan into action.

The energy plan is not about losing weight, although many people will experience some weight loss. The goal is to get rid of the many foods and behaviors surrounding us that sap our energy. The food-energy sappers induce an inflammatory state and abdominal weight gain and they increase hunger and cravings because they spike blood sugar followed by insulin release, leaving you unsatisfied.

If you experience weight loss it only represents elimination of calories from these foods. But my Everyday Energy Plan is not about deprivation. In fact, the energy zappers deprive the body of health, vitality, and vigor. My plan restores your natural energetic state. You will have to refuse 90 percent of the snack foods that you will be offered, because it will zap your energy and drag you down. But that doesn't mean you can't snack; you just have to be selective. And in this plan, there are great healthy snacking ideas. For example, just say no to the morning bagel or doughnut, to the plates of cookies in the coffee room at work, to the ubiquitous candy around Christmas, to the bread basket, to diet or sugary sodas, to sitting in front of the TV with a bag of chips, pretzels, or Oreos, which you mindlessly consume. But do say yes to a crunchy green apple or a slice of freshly made low-fat mozzarella.

DO I NEED TO COUNT CALORIES?

All my patients ask me this when they embark on my plan. In a word, *no*, you do not need to count calories, points, or carbs. By the way, in my clinical practice I never design a diet based on calories alone. All calories are not the same; different foods have different effects within the body as I have explained. I have seen far too many people who limit their calories without regard to the nutritional content of the food. It is the nutrition that matters. Do not count calories. Instead focus on the nutritional value of the food.

THE GUARDIAN

Think of yourself as an armed guard. You have been armed with knowledge of nutrition and your job is to guard your health. You are the guardian of your own health. No uninvited intruders are allowed by the guard (you). The guard always asks, "What benefit does it have to health?" Only foods that benefit health are allowed in. Continuing with this analogy: At a cocktail party, you are offered a doughy hors d'oeuvre. . . . Does it have any benefit to health? No. It is not allowed in. Next you are offered a cocktail shrimp. . . . Does it have any benefit to health? Yes. It is high in lean protein and will benefit your health. While working you become hungry before a meal, do you chose a handful of almonds or a bag of chips? Which of these benefits your health? The guard must always ask the benefit to health. The energy plan is a proactive approach to health.

SIX BASIC ENERGY PRINCIPLES

---

1. Begin every day with a protein-packed breakfast. It will keep you satisfied longer. Morning protein sources are: omega-3 eggs, turkey bacon, yogurt, cheese, cottage cheese, smoked salmon, fish, or chicken.
2. Include protein at every meal and snack. Protein will keep you satisfied longer and allows your body to renew itself.
3. Drink ten glasses of water daily. Bottled flat or sparkling, or plain tap water with a squeeze of fruit. Avoid sweetened waters.

4. Eat a big salad every day to give yourself a good supply of the power molecules.

5. Exercise every single day of your life. Mornings are best. If you are alive, you should be moving.

6. Coffee and tea are fine. By all means enjoy them in the morning, but try to hold off consuming them in the afternoon as they may interfere with sleep.

RISE AND SHINE "TAKE-ALONG" BREAKFASTS

There are times when everyone needs to grab something for breakfast and run out the door. Just because you are in a rush doesn't mean you must sacrifice a healthy start to your day. Below are quick and simple but nutritious starts to the day that I recommend to my patients.

- *Hard-Boiled Omega-3 Egg*—A hard-boiled omega-3 egg has 8g protein and 150mg omega-3 fat. Don't worry about the cholesterol in that egg— the omega-3 fat cancels it out! An orange will add vitamin C. (If you work in an office, I suggest boiling a few eggs on the weekends so you don't have to bother on weekday mornings.)

- *Light n' Lively Cottage Cheese*—Calcium-enriched product that is high in protein. Add some strawberries for power molecules and vitamin C. Cottage cheese is high in protein but low in calcium. Light n' Lively adds calcium to their cottage cheese.

- *Fage, Brown Cow, and Stonyfield Farm Yogurt*—Fat-free yogurts are sources of protein and calcium. Buy the plain fat-free variety and add your own fruit: in summer, berries or peaches or plums or cherries. In winter, serve it with a baked pear or a baked apple with cinnamon. Or take a Ziploc bag with whole grain cereal and stir it into a carton of yogurt.

- *Omega-3 Enriched Yogurt with Fruit*—Switch to omega-3 enriched yogurt topped with sliced green apples and sprinkle with a teaspoon of wheat germ.

- *My Everyday Nutrition Ready-to-Drink Shake*—The shake is rich and high in protein, omega-3s, and calcium. It is satisfying and suppresses hunger naturally.

THINK OUTSIDE OF THE BOX (OF CEREAL)

Although a slice of turkey on whole grain bread, for example, isn't a traditional breakfast food, no one would disparage you for eating one at 8 A.M. Some of my patients even have their dinner leftovers for breakfast! How about a breakfast burrito of grilled chicken, low-fat Monterey Jack cheese, salsa, and mango? My own favorite breakfast is smoked salmon and melon with fresh lemon and ground pepper. The important thing is to see your breakfast as something you do for yourself to benefit your health. If you want to do your best work and feel energetic, you *must* eat breakfast!

DR. KLAUER'S FAVORITE BREAKFAST GRAINS

- Kashi GOLEAN
- McCann's Oatmeal
- Uncle Sam's Toasted Whole Grain Wheat Flakes
- Arrowhead Mills hot and cold Cereals—7 Grain Hot Cereal is a favorite in my home. All their cereals are organic and kosher. Look for 4g or more of fiber.

SAMPLE MENU PLAN

DAY I—

Breakfast: Energy Omelet, page 178, of two large omega-3 eggs with I ounce low-fat cheese, I tablespoon onion, ¼ cup chopped red pepper, and a handful of chopped fresh parsley or cilantro.

Lunch: Arugula salad with shaved Parmesan cheese. Grilled wild salmon with lemon.

Snack: Fresh veggie sticks (carrots, celery, yellow peppers) with guacamole.

Dinner: Ginger Soy Chicken, page 178, wild rice, green beans amandine. After dinner a cup of ginger tea will assist digestion.

Energy bullet: Ginger *(Zingiber officinale)* is a spice that dates back more than three thousand years. Native to Asia, ginger is a staple in many Asian dishes and is used to treat digestive disturbances. Research now confirms that the antioxidant polyphenol gingerol, found in the gingerroot, is responsible for the medicinal effects. Studies suggest that ginger is a go-to for motion sickness, nausea, indigestion, and can ease inflammatory conditions like arthritis. To brew ginger tea, place several slices of fresh ginger in a tea strainer and steep in boiling water for 5 to 8 minutes. The fresh gingerroot should be stored unwrapped in your refrigerator.

DAY 2—

Breakfast: Yogurt Energy Starter, page 177.

Lunch: Mandarin orange, walnut, and spinach salad, grilled shrimp.

Snack: One apple (the top variety for antioxidants is Red Delicious) and 2 ounces low-fat Muenster cheese. If you can't eat cheese, have 3 to 4 ounces of chicken or a 4-ounce can of tuna in its place. You could even have hummus, and substitute crudités for the apple with any of these proteins.

Dinner: Grilled wild Alaskan salmon, asparagus, and wild rice.

◎Energy bullet: Wild king salmon from Alaska offers 1000mg omega-3 fat per serving. Omega-3 fat benefits the health of heart and mind. By consuming the salmon and asparagus at the same meal the fat soluble vitamins A and K (present in the asparagus) are absorbed more readily. Fat soluble vitamins require fat for absorption. Omega-3 helps your body to absorb the vitamins. At lunch, the walnuts on the salad contain omega-3 fat in the plant form, alpha linolenic acid (ALA). The ALA present in the walnuts helps your body to absorb the fat soluble vitamins A, E, and K present in the spinach and the vitamin D in the cheese. Omega-3 fat, in both fish and plants, boosts energy by helping fat soluble vitamins enter your body.

DAY 3—

Breakfast: High-Energy Berry Blast, page 177.

Lunch: Grilled trout with lemon and capers. Broiled tomato-eggplant slices drizzled with basil oil.

Snack: Vegetable crudités with olives and Parmigiano-Reggiano cheese.

Dinner: Buffalo kebabs with tomato, portobello mushrooms, and zucchini. Quinoa with pine nuts.

⑤Energy bullet: If you have never had buffalo meat, you are in for a treat! Buffalo or bison is considered the new red meat. It is leaner than beef, and even chicken, and contains 40 percent more protein than beef. The fat that it does have contains omega-3 fat and has a healthier profile than commercially raised beef, which has more saturated fat. Bison is said to have a sweeter, richer flavor than beef. It is high in niacin, vitamins B6 and B12, and selenium. Like all meats it contains no carbohydrate and is high in protein. Bison is a deeper red color than beef before cooking because there is no marbling—those white flecks of fat within the meat muscle. Remember when you cook buffalo meat, use lower heat and moisture-retaining techniques. Searing buffalo meat on both sides helps to seal in the natural juices. It will cook faster than beef.

MEATS	FATS	CALORIES	CHOLESTEROL	SATURATED FAT
BISON	2.42g	143 cal	82mg	0.91g
BEEF	9.91g	216 cal	86mg	3.79g
CHICKEN	7.41g	190 cal	89mg	2.04g

Source: www.arrowheadsteaks.com; figures are for 100g of cooked lean meat

One of my patients, Eden, was on holiday in Rome with her teenage daughter. She was conscious of sticking with her Energy Plan and not coming back with extra pounds from gelato and pasta. So she asked the concierge at her hotel to recommend a wonderful Roman restaurant. He chose his personal favorite—a little-known place with only eight tables in one of the winding cobblestoned streets near Piazza Navona. They walked and walked to find it, which made them build up an appetite as well as give them some added exercise. Finally, there was a tap on Eden's shoulder, from a gentleman in a white apron saying *Scusi,* who assumed they were the Americans sent from Hotel Gladiatori. It turned out that the restaurant's signature dishes were all made from buffalo, including fresh buffalo mozzarella, buffalo prime rib, lasagna bisonese, and homemade buffalo sausage. Eden said it was the best meal they had in Italy!

DAY 4—Breakfast: Caviar omelet with a side order of blueberries.
Lunch: Selenium Salad, page 180. Field greens with grilled tuna and slivered Brazil nuts. (Tuna and Brazil nuts are two of the highest natural selenium foods known.)
Snack: One sliced white nectarine with a handful of almonds.
Dinner: Ginger-steamed cod with bok choy and scallions. Wild rice with lemon zest.

◎ Energy bullet: Selenium is a mineral that has been linked to energy and health. Within the body selenium forms complexes with proteins called selenoproteins, which regulate our immune system. Selenium is present in the soil and deficiencies occur only in regions where the selenium of the soil is low. Lunch today included the two highest sources of natural selenium: tuna and Brazil nuts. A recent study showed that selenium in the diet helps keep your muscles strong.[1]

Selenium also can be found in seafood such as cod. Animals such as cows, turkeys, and chicken that eat grains or plants, which were grown in selenium-rich soil, have higher levels of selenium in their muscles.

DAY 5—Breakfast: Two scrambled eggs with red and yellow peppers and part-skim mozzarella cheese. One side order of blueberries.
Lunch: Spiced Shrimp with Cucumber Salad, page 179. Sliced tomatoes on the side.
Snack: One cup fat-free plain yogurt with raspberries.
Dinner: Organic free-range filet mignon grilled with herbs. Roasted Sweet Potato Fries, page 187, and spinach.

◎ Energy bullet: Sweet potatoes are high in the antioxidant beta carotene. Unlike white potatoes, they do not spike the blood sugar, even though they taste mildly sweet. Sweet potatoes are an excellent source of fiber, vitamins A and C, and some calcium. The recipe for Roasted Sweet Potato Fries (page 187) is a favorite of my family's.

DAY 6—Breakfast: Sunrise Chicken Quesadilla, page 177, with mango salsa.
Lunch: Salad Niçoise with seared tuna.
Snack: One apple and a handful of walnuts.
Dinner: Broiled lobster with lemon, parsley, and summer squash.

ⓖEnergy bullet: Think outside of the griddle. Beginning your day with a
quesadilla may seem a bit unusual, but my recipe will supply you with
high protein, calcium, antioxidants, and the fiber you need.

DAY 7—Breakfast: I cup cottage cheese and ½ cup mixed berries with 3
tablespoons chopped walnuts.
Lunch: Grilled wild Alaskan salmon with white asparagus with citrus zest.
Snack: One apple and one organic part-skim mozzarella stick.
Dinner: Dinner salad with Alaskan halibut and papaya.

ⓖEnergy bullet: Day-seven meals have over 2,200mg omega-3 fat.
Omega-3 fat protects the heart and brain from oxidative damage
through anti-inflammatory mechanisms. The membranes of cells within
the brain and nervous system contain the highest concentrations of
omega-3 fat of the entire body. If energy is your goal, it is just common
sense to build a strong foundation of healthy brain cells with omega-3 fat.
See page 178 for Ginger Soy Chicken and page 179 for Spiced
Shrimp with Cucumber Salad.

MONOSODIUM GLUTAMATE (MSG)

While shopping for chicken broth I noted that many of the broths on the
shelf did not contain MSG. I found this to be surprising as MSG is used as a traditional, if controversial, flavor enhancer. But after quick Web-based research, it
turns out that the U.S. Food and Drug Administration requires manufacturers to
list MSG only if it is in its pure form. But many food additives contain glutamate
and may be included without the special labeling: autolyzed yeast, yeast extract,
dried whey, hydrolyzed soy protein, and disodium inosinate. Even more surprising is that the labels on many of the products containing these additives proudly
announce "No MSG." If you are sensitive to MSG, be sure to look at labels for
any of the above compounds. There is a lot of hidden MSG out there, especially
in foods for children, and many parents do not realize this. Chinese restaurants in

America often print right on their menus "Our foods do not contain MSG." You can also specifically ask for your food to be cooked without MSG.

> The best chicken broth is the one you make yourself—your own home-made chicken broth with organic chicken, celery, onions, carrots, and fresh herbs. (See Maggie Ella's Good-for-You Chicken Soup recipe, originally from my grandmother on page 188.) If you do not have the time or inclination to make your own, try these: Swanson's Certified Organic Free-Range Chicken Broth, Imagine Organic Free-Range Chicken Broth. As a substitute, you can also use your own vegetable broth. (See Very Veggie Consommé on page 181).

ON-THE-RUN MEALS

I understand that there are times when you will not be able to sit down at a table to consume a leisurely meal. But when this time arises, if you have prepared ahead you won't have a problem. An Everyday Nutrition shake is the perfect quick energy fix on the go.

Planning ahead and preparing a healthy meal is another strategy. The important idea is to be mindful of the food that you consume. If you don't plan ahead, you may get caught without a healthy option available.

BREAKFAST ON THE RUN—Breakfast should never be just a bagel or a Danish with coffee. Doughy food will make you doughy. By all means drink your coffee, but include protein for lasting energy. Below are high-protein examples that have worked for my patients.

- Everyday Nutrition shake
- Fat-free plain yogurt. Add one luscious, ripened organic peach. Ten almonds or pistachios in a bag.
- 1 hard-boiled omega-3 egg with 2 ounces of cheese and a medium-sized Bartlett pear.
- 1 cup low-fat ricotta cheese with ground cinnamon, ½ cup blueberries, a sprinkling of pistachio nuts.
- Omega-3 egg salad with five Kashi TLC crackers and one apple.

LUNCH ON THE RUN—Is lunch your downfall? Many people end up skipping lunch entirely because there is nothing healthy available. Still many others eat the wrong things and feel guilty for the rest of the day because they strayed from their plan.

When you are busy it is tempting just to skip a meal and keep going. On an energy level, this is robbing Peter to pay Paul! It doesn't work. During the crunch times it is even more important to eat in a healthy manner. Don't fall into the fast food habit. By preparing your own lunch you can improve on even the healthiest fast food options.

Take your lunch along:

- Everyday Nutrition shake with one piece of fresh fruit.
- Whole wheat tortilla with fresh arugula, avocado slices, tomato slices, and roast chicken. One piece of fruit.
- One four-ounce pop-top can of dark Italian tuna with Ziploc bag of crudités of fresh vegetables and olives.
- Lentil soup or turkey chili in a thermos. Whole grain crackers and 2 to 3 ounces low-fat cheese. One piece of fruit: apple, pear, or peach.
- Salmon Croquettes (page 180) on salad of red leaf lettuce, cucumbers, and dill. One piece of fruit: apple, pear, or peach.

DINNER—Europeans eat their main meal midday, so for dinner, they eat later and lighter than Americans do. We tend not to dine; we are a nation of grazers. Families don't often sit down with their children anymore.

For starters, it is better to eat earlier rather than later. Dinner should be a healthful meal that is consumed with your family and friends, which reinforces your commitment to the principles of good nutrition for your children.

Gastroesophageal reflux is caused by people going to bed with too much food in their stomach. The force of gravity is pushing down on the stomach contents while the tension of a full stomach is pulling the sphincter. Two different forces are acting on the sphincter, causing acid to escape. We experience this as heartburn, which can damage the cells of the esophagus. Other things that cause the sphincter to be lax are alcohol and chocolate. So by having a smaller dinner earlier and avoiding alcohol, you will feel better and sleep better, too.

DINNER ON THE RUN—Dinner on the run could be when you are buried in the office getting paperwork done for a morning meeting. Or when you are in-between flights and stuck in an airport for hours. Or when you are trying to squeeze in a meal before going to the theater for an eight o'clock curtain. We all find ourselves in these situations once in a while. For some, it can be quite often. Here are some of the tips I suggest for healthy quick dinners in these situations.

TAKEOUT AT THE OFFICE—Instead of ordering lo mein from the nearest Chinese takeout, try ordering steamed chicken and broccoli and avoid the egg rolls. Another good alternative from the local pizza place is a Greek salad. From the local coffee shop try a chicken wrap with vegetables—it can be a lighter option, but hold the mayo. And always avoid French fries!

AIRPORT DINING—Most airports have a few restaurants that are open at all hours and serve breakfast food 24/7. One good omega-3 enriched meal could be scrambled eggs with a side of vegetables or a salad. This meal is light enough so it won't weigh you down when you are running for your gate, and it won't spike your sugar sky-high either.

AIRPORT A-TEAM—If you are stuck between flights, here are some of my best bets for hungry travelers. Watch out for added sodium, high-fat entrées, and anything called "crispy," which means it is fried or battered. Also make sure to get sauce or dressing on the side.

- Sbarro—Pass up the heavy pasta, pizza, and garlic bread, and go for the Greek salad.
- T.G.I. Friday's—Jack Daniel's Shrimp and Salmon, but ask for a vegetable substitute for the mashed potatoes, such as steamed broccoli.
- Chili's—Stick with the Guiltless Grill choices, but stay away from baked potatoes and fries.
- Wendy's—Mandarin Chicken Salad is probably your lightest option.
- McDonald's—Premium salads offer greener choices, and the Chipotle Barbecued Snack Wrap with Grilled Chicken is a good one.

COCKTAILS AFTER WORK?

If you are going for a drink after work, and you have no food in your stomach, the alcohol will go to your head quickly. Instead of munching on salty pretzels, ask for some nuts or order a light appetizer such as crudités, cheese, skewered chicken, or a shrimp cocktail. Order a bottle of mineral water for hydration, then one cocktail.

PHASE TWO—YOUR NEW PLAN FOR AN ENERGETIC LIFE

Now that you have committed yourself to a healthy lifestyle and thrown away the foods that undermine health, it is time to loosen up the reins of Phase One. The purpose of Phase One is to eliminate many of the foods frequently consumed in the American diet that deplete energy. Take a look around you: Do the people you see look vibrant and energetic? I suspect the answer is "no." Many people simply accept their increasing lethargy as part of the aging process or attribute it to stress brought about from others. Both of these explanations are untrue and demonstrate passive acceptance of an unnecessary condition. In fact, we all can control our health and we are able to prevent the majority of disease.

Our elegantly designed bodies can take an enormous amount of abuse but today in the United States we are pushing the limit. With all our great wealth, we have centered our lives on inactivity and consumption of food with minimal nutritional value. The extent of the damage that we are doing to ourselves is evident from the recent announcement that the U.S. life expectancy has now fallen to forty-first in the world. As you have eliminated overly processed food and inactivity you have taken the road of health and energy. You will feel energetic because your body is fueled with the foods associated with health.

Phase Two is the plan that you follow for life. Take care as you add more food to the plan. If you begin to feel tired or your alertness begins to sink, step back and assess what foods might have triggered this. You have seen very clearly how eating right and exercising can revitalize you. Now your goal should be to keep on feeling great.

The first food to add will be grains. Grains are important as they supply fiber and nutrients. Make sure that you are adding whole grains. Keep avoiding refined wheat flour: it offers no benefit to your body. (Remember, you're the guardian of your health!)

Whole grains benefit your digestive system. They provide fiber and reduce your risk for developing heart disease and diabetes. Refined flour increases your risk for diabetes.

BREAKFAST

Protein in the morning will keep you from feeling hungry until lunch. If you want to add a slice of whole grain toast, be my guest. A breakfast with a good amount of protein and high-fiber carbohydrate will keep you satisfied because it will gradually raise blood glucose and insulin. Build your breakfast around protein, starting with eggs, yogurt, cheese, etc., and then add either cereal or toast. If you are having cereal, skip the toast as you are carb-loading at that point. If you have a rough time controlling your weight, I strongly suggest that you hold off on starchy food for breakfast.

In Phase One you eliminated fruit that ranked high on the glycemic index. By doing so you avoided a hunger-provoking insulin spike. Although bananas, grapes, and pineapples are higher glycemic fruits, instead of eating them on their own, they can make a good addition to high-protein smoothies. Use a small ripe banana or half a ripe regular banana to thicken the smoothie. Bananas, grapes, and pineapples should be combined with a serving of protein. See my recipes for breakfast smoothies (page 177).

You eliminated juices in Phase One and I encourage you to continue avoiding them. By drinking juice, you are missing out on the fiber of the whole fruit and the power molecules contained in the skin of the fruit. Stay away from drinking juices and keep eating the whole fruit instead. But feel free to use fruit juices in cooking to supply sweetness.

PHASE TWO—Breakfast Additions

- Whole grain toast
- Whole grain cereals
- Whole grain waffle or pancake as a weekend treat
- Banana and pineapple may be added to smoothies or cottage cheese.

LUNCH AND DINNER

During lunch and dinner in Phase One you avoided bread while decid-ing what to order. If you wish to occasionally include bread before a meal then do so mindfully. I suggest that you form the habit of asking for olive oil with the bread and avoid the high-saturated-fat butter. Recognize that the bread is a food from grain and may be overly processed and refined or it may be whole grain. Whole grain bread benefits the digestion because of fiber and vitamins contained in the bran and germ layers. Take a good look at the bread you are considering and if it is not a whole grain bread leave it alone.

Test your bread. How do you find out if your bread is made from whole grains? Look for visible fibers and you should not be able to form it into a ball.

What about rice, potatoes, and pasta? Using the same line of reasoning as you used with bread, analyze what you are going to consume. Rice is a grain and may be either whole grain—as in brown rice—or refined white rice. Stick with brown rice. Cooked brown rice contains 5g protein and 4g fiber; white rice contains 4g protein and no fiber. Get into the habit of requesting brown rice. I prefer the more full-bodied taste, and you will too. It is small changes like this that begin to make a difference in your health.

Pasta can also be whole grain or refined. Both plain and spinach pasta have only 3g protein and 0g fiber. Whole wheat pasta typically has 7.5g protein and 3.9g fiber per one cup cooked. Make whole wheat pasta your choice. Whole wheat pastas are firmer with a slightly "nutty" flavor and are a superior choice nutritionally. White potatoes are fine occasionally, but please don't have them every night. (Sweet potatoes contain more fiber and power molecules; enjoy them as often as you wish.)

Wine has a benefit to health, but drinking wine to excess will hurt you. Wine can be a complement to a good meal, relaxing us and allowing us to sa-vor the tastes and moment. But drinking too much wine makes us intoxicated. My advice: Drink a glass or two and that is all.

WHOLE WHEAT PASTA

Try Eden Organic 100% Whole Grain Pasta—Take your pick from rigatoni, spaghetti, gemelli, and spirals; they have many delicious and nutritious varieties to choose from. www.edenfoods.com

Did you know that many restaurants today will substitute brown rice for white rice in sushi? Just get in the habit of asking the waiter when you place your order.

PHASE TWO—Lunch and Dinner Additions

- Brown rice
- Whole wheat pasta
- Whole grain bread (dip into olive oil)
- White potatoes occasionally
- Wine occasionally

SANDWICHES THAT SIZZLE—Sandwiches are pretty standard lunch fare, but you can keep it healthy and interesting. Instead of the usual boring sandwich of a few slices of meat stuffed between two slices of white bread, try something with color, texture, and flavor to wake up your taste buds!

- Whole wheat pita pockets. "Stone ground whole wheat flour, water, salt, yeast, malted barley flour, and calcium propionate (added to retard spoilage)." This is a great list of ingredients for bread. There is no refined flour to be found here. If you use a four- or five-inch pita you will save approximately a hundred calories over a sandwich made with two slices of doughy bread. Toast lightly, or even throw it on the grill when you can to add some crunch.
- Wraps or tortillas made with one hundred percent whole wheat. Some of my favorite brands include:
  - South Beach Diet Wraps—multigrain or whole wheat
  - Thomas Sahara Wraps—one hundred percent whole wheat

- Flatout Wraps—one hundred percent stone ground whole wheat
- La Tortilla Factory Carb Cutting Low-Fat Organic Wheat Tortillas

DESSERTS IN PHASE TWO

Of the four tastes (sour, salty, sweet, and bitter) only sweet has an entire meal course dedicated to it. We should enjoy desserts, just not every night. Moderation has to be the key with desserts because they taste so good. The idea is not denial so much as to be thoughtful about the food you consume. Any dessert may be eaten in moderation. If it is the custom in your family to have dessert, make it fruit.

Each Christmas dinner in our family ends with a spectacular dessert prepared by my husband. In fact, the dessert has become so popular that our family and friends begin talking about it in the fall. At the end of our Christmas dinner and after the exchange of gifts, our dining room is bathed in soft candlelight—this perfectly sets the stage for my husband to make his entrance through the dining room doors with a large silver tray bearing a beautiful Baked Alaska. The small children (and adults) are transfixed by the magic of his lighting the dessert, watching the flaming meringues, and then being served a piece of the delicious concoction. The sugar and ice cream contained in the extravagant creation is a memorable indulgence for all. It says, " 'Tis the season to be jolly!"

I include this story because I want you to realize that there are occasions like this where the moment does take over, and indulgence is warranted. But if you are taking care of yourself by eating in a healthy manner, you can relax and indulge with nary a thought of the consequences. (And definitely get yourself on the treadmill the next morning.)

THREE-DAY MINI DETOX ENERGIZING PROGRAM

We've all been there: those times when you really let go and your diet goes to hell in a handbasket. Christmas holidays, a big party you are giving, a food and wine weekend—all can sap your energy and leave you exhausted. These things happen. What matters is not that they happen but what you are going to do about it.

This three-day plan is for times when you just need to get back on track. First, the mini detox energizing program eliminates the foods that were responsible for the energy slump. No alcohol. Throw or give away leftovers. Begin by increasing your water consumption, because it has probably fallen. (The first thing I notice when someone falls off their diet is that they have stopped religiously drinking two to three liters of water daily.) Resolve to go to the gym every day.

On the mini detox plan variety is limited, but it is for only three days. I have found people do better with limited choices when they are stressed. The foods listed have strong nutritional benefit and will renew your vitality.

DETOX DAYS—Begin each day with a big glass of water, and go to the gym for one hour. Avoid sugar in any form in your diet for three days to rid your body of bloat. Eliminate processed foods and alcohol. Drink two to three liters of water daily. Be sure to eat every four hours.

Breakfast: I cup plain, fat-free yogurt with ½ cup organic berries. Coffee or tea.

Lunch: Lots of greens. A big salad with dark green lettuce, spinach, or arugula. Add tomato, carrot, cucumber, asparagus, peppers, and red onion. Dress your salad with I tablespoon olive oil and a splash of vinegar. Choose one of the following proteins with the salad: grilled salmon, tuna, red snapper, sea bass, or shrimp. Drink mineral water with lemon or lime.

Snack: I cup of plain, fat-free yogurt with raw vegetables, I cup green tea. Continue drinking water throughout the afternoon.

Dinner: Grilled fish with herbs, a side salad, and two servings of vegetables (one should be green). Fresh berries for dessert, followed by decaffeinated green tea or herbal tea.

LIVING THE SPA LIFE

Let's face it—every busy person needs a little more spa in their life! Keeping up your energy is also about finding ways to relax and having downtime.

THREE GREAT ENERGY BOOSTERS

1. Swedish massage
2. Shiatsu massage
3. Sauna—Followed by a dip in the pool.

PERFECT WEEKEND REWIND

There are times in everyone's life when you may feel like you are going to hit a wall if you don't get away. I encourage my clients to take advantage of the replenishing effects of a weekend away from work, kids, partners, and the daily stress of life at home. The best way to do that is to get on a train, plane, or in a car and go somewhere to change your scenery. You will be amazed at how even two or three days in a new place can perk up your spirits and restore your energy level.

These are two of my favorites:

- Miraval, Tucson, Arizona—An amazing sprawling facility where the emphasis is on getting life back into balance. They don't push their own products or medical treatments, and they provide exceptional care and pampering. www.miravalresort.com
- Mayflower Inn & Spa, Washington, Connecticut—A luxury five-star retreat just a few hours from the hustle and bustle of New York City. www.mayflowerinn.com
- The Canyon Ranch, Lenox, Massachusetts—The tranquil setting offers a variety of energizing exercise classes and superb lectures about health.

CHAPTER SIX

POWER MOLECULES IN FOOD

Tell me what you eat, and I will tell you what you are.

—ANTHELME BRILLAT-SAVARIN

Always think about your goal: higher energy and good health.

Our goal in eating should be to give ourselves the best in nutrition. We need to be not just reactive to foods that are presented to us; we must be proactive in feeding ourselves. Having a diet containing the power molecules allows the body to repair and renew itself.

WHAT ARE POWER MOLECULES?

Scientific research is now focusing on newly identified color pigments in plants. Beyond the vitamins and minerals found in plants we eat are the pigment power molecules that offer extra benefits to the body. Power molecules are exciting because of their abundance. Most people realize that vegetables and fruits contain vitamins, but they might not be aware of the power molecules. Basically the power molecules are the pigments that give color to plants. The colorful pigments are referred to as phytochemicals, from the Greek root, "phyto" for plant. Nature seems to have a reason for every-thing and that is true for the phytochemicals. Phytochemicals protect the plant from the UV radiation in sunlight, fight off insects by scent, or at-tract insects by color; in short the phytochemicals are responsible for the plants' survival. These wonderful substances have always been present in plants and we are only now identifying the many thousands of phyto-chemicals and researching their functions. If you keep your meals colorful with a variety of vegetables and fruit, you will be rewarded with renewed energy and health.

EVERYDAY FOOD

There are foods that you should eat daily to keep your energy high and your health in top form.

- *Berries.* All types of berries are high in antioxidants. Blueberries have high amounts of resveratrol and flavonoids. Strawberries and raspberries are high in vitamin C.
- *Leafy green vegetables.* The greener, the better. Vegetables, a power-house of vitamins, and green leafy vegetables have omega-3 fat. Spinach, kale, purslane, etc.
- *Yogurt.* Promotes growth of healthy bacteria in the intestines, im-proves motility, and reduces the risk for colon polyps.
- *Fish.* Contains lean protein and supplies omega-3 fatty acids.
- *Whole grains.* Whole grains supply fiber, vitamins, and minerals. Look for whole wheat pasta.
- *Tea.* Herbal teas, green, white, and black teas contain EGCG—a power molecule in the flavonoid family.
- *Olive oil.* High-quality olive oil should be your choice in preparing meals. Grilled vegetables and meats are enhanced by a light coat-ing. Olive oil helps to lower the dangerous LDL cholesterol.
- *Nuts.* Nuts contain power molecules and minerals. The fat in nuts will not raise your cholesterol.

Within the past few years nutritional science has identified molecules found naturally in familiar foods that contain true benefit for the body. The effects of the power molecules include improved memory, lower risk for heart attacks, better eyesight, and reduced risk for certain cancers and longer life. While many of the names are unusual (some difficult to pronounce) we would be wise to commit the foods to memory and incorporate them into our diets. Most of what is known about the benefits of vitamins relates to the vitamin as found in food.

BASIC FOOD GROUPS PLUS POWER MOLECULES

You already know that vegetables and fruits are natural sources for vitamins. Many vitamins work as antioxidants, meaning they repair damage we incur just by living. Some work as cofactors to important components of metabolic cycles. For example, the process of blood forming a clot is dependent on vitamin E and vitamin C. Without the two vitamins we would bleed to death from the slightest injury. Vitamin E and C have other important functions and also act as antioxidants.

GO GOJI!

Wolfberries or *Goji* berries are now grown around the world, primarily in China and Tibet. They have been used in traditional Eastern medicine for centuries. These potent little berries are loaded with antioxidants, and you can pick these up in dried varieties or in liquid form as a juice at your natural grocery or health food store. Add them to smoothies, fruit salads, soups, and vegetables dishes.

Not all vitamins are antioxidants. But all vitamins perform vital functions in our body. The power molecules (polyphenols and phytochemicals) have benefits above and beyond antioxidants and vitamins.

Vitamin	Health Benefits
• A—5000 IU	(Beta carotene) Vision, eyes, clear skin, healthy bones, hair, teeth.
• B_1—1.5mg	(Thiamin) Nervous system, appetite, energy, nerve conduction.
• B_{12}—6mcg	For the blood: Prevents pernicious anemia, important for healthy nervous system, directly involved in synthesis of genetic material (DNA).
• B_2—1.7mg	(Riboflavin) For skin, eyes, energy.
• B_3—20mg	(Niacin) For the skin, nervous system, and mental performance.
• B_5—10mg	(Pantothenic acid) Develops acetylcholine, a neurotransmitter. Synthesis of fatty acids for membranes, cholesterol, hormones.
• B_6—2mg	Helps metabolize protein and fat, needed for red blood cells and hemoglobin synthesis.
• Biotin—0.30mg	Metabolizes amino acids, hair growth, strong nails.
• C—60mg	Antioxidant that builds up the immune system to prevent colds and illnesses, minimizes the effects of free radicals and nitrosamines related to carcinogens. Structural element in skin and bones.
• Choline	Prevents fat accumulation in the liver, neurotransmitter in the brain.
• D—400 IU	Calcium and phosphorus metabolism for strong bones and teeth. Healthy immune system. Note level is under investigation currently; my advice is over age forty years, consume eight hundred IU/day. If you are not in the sun daily, ask your doctor to measure your level.
• E—30 IU	Prevents oxidation of proteins, fats, and vitamin A, protects red blood cells. Health of nervous system.
• Folic Acid—0.4mg	Red blood cell formation, metabolizes fats, amino acids, protein synthesis, DNA synthesis.
• Inositol	Involved in calcium mobilization.
• K	Helps the blood clot properly.

In addition to vitamins, nutritional science is now directed toward an exciting group of power molecules, the polyphenols. The power molecules occur naturally in all vegetables and fruits. We are discovering new power molecules all the time. These mighty molecules give protection to heart, brain, and against cancer. Additionally, polyphenols, as the active constituent of medicinal plants, have specific biological properties, most of which we are just beginning to understand. One of the reasons why clinical nutrition is so exciting to me is the new research that seems to uncover the benefits of plants in the diet. The power molecules may be divided into two groups: the carotenoids and flavonoids.

Antioxidant vitamins, such as *carotenoids*, neutralize free radicals in the body. *Lutein* promotes healthy vision. *Lycopene* may decrease the risk for certain types of cancer. A variety of plant compounds called *flavonols*,—including *anthocyanins* and *catechins*—halt damage from free radicals.

CAROTENOIDS

These are natural fat-soluble pigments in plants, algae, and photosynthetic bacteria, where they are essential for photosynthesis. Each color has a particular type of property. For instance, the red pigment in tomatoes, lycopene, protects against prostate cancer. Beta carotene, an orange pigment, is found in carrots. The most well-defined function of the carotenoids is its provitamin A activity, necessary for vision. Vitamin A is produced within our body when we consume the carotenoids found in carrots, sweet potatoes, spinach, apricots, and other sources. Sight occurs because of a chemical reaction within the retina requiring vitamin A. In addition to antioxidant actions, our eyesight depends on carotenoids. It is important to note that the carotenoids are fat soluble. The carotenoids are best absorbed from food when fat is present in the meal. This doesn't mean putting a glob of butter on your sweet potato! But for the best absorption, include olive oil in the meal and top your sweet potato with chopped walnuts—which contain healthful fat.

The process by which we see is quite extraordinary. Vision is something that we take for granted but how we perceive our environment is an astonishing process. The eye has two types of photosensitive cells: rods and cones. Both cells are unlike any other cells in the body as far as their shape is concerned; while other neurons have a cell body and appendages that project to adjacent cells, the rods and cones possess minute invaginations of their cellular membranes on one side of their membranes to capture light. Picture a rat-tail comb—that's how they look! Cones are responsible for day vision; people who lose cone function are legally blind. Cones allow color vision and provide detail. There are three basic types of cone cells, allowing us to tell the difference between yellow, blue, and red.

Rods are responsible for night vision; they function in dim light, when the light is too weak to stimulate the cones. Total loss of rods produces only night blindness. Light activates a visual pigment within the photosensitive cell. The visual pigment that absorbs light is retinal, a form of vitamin A. In the dark, the retina fits snugly in a coiled position; when light hits it a change in shape occurs. The change occurs in a fraction of a second, and then it flips back to the original shape. The conformational change activates a cascade of events that results in the signal traveling to the brain via the optic nerve.

Think of it! The morning light, newspaper, faces of loved ones, our computer screens, etc., are all recognizable because of intricate processing with our eyes. This incredible process is dependent on vitamin A.

KEY CAROTENOIDS

- Lutein
- Zeaxanthin

Lutein and zeaxanthin are found in highest concentration in green leafy plants. In plants, lutein and zeaxanthin protect the chloroplast (think of this as the heart of the plant) from damage from blue light. These power molecules protect our eyes by reducing free radical damage. As we age our eyes are vulnerable to cataracts (clouded lens) and macular degeneration (breakdown of the center of the retina). The protective powers of lutein and zeaxanthin were suspected when researchers found that carotenoids concentrate in the eye. In fact, the concentrations of lutein and zeaxanthin are one hundred times higher in the macula than in the blood. In both lens and retina they act as antioxidants. But within the retina they also act as a filter that protects the macula by absorbing short-wavelength light, which is toxic to the retina. Think of them as internal sunglasses.

In several large studies, it has been found that people who consume the most lutein and zeaxanthin had a 20 to 50 percent lower risk of cataracts.[1, 2] Studies have also found that the risk of macular degeneration is lowered by eating lutein and zeaxanthin.[3, 4]

The best way to obtain these power molecules is from eating leafy vegetables. Not only do the leafy vegetables supply fiber, vitamins C, K, and A, but they are a natural source of high amounts of lutein and zeaxanthin. Just by including a daily salad, you may head off vision loss.

ARE YOU AT RISK FOR MACULAR DEGENERATION?

- Age is a risk. Macular degeneration is the leading cause of severe vision loss after age sixty.
- Macular degeneration may be hereditary. If you have relatives with the condition you are at higher risk for developing the condition.
- Smoking causes constriction of the blood vessels and is a major risk factor.

WHAT ARE THE SYMPTOMS OF MACULAR DEGENERATION?

- Straight lines appear wavy as the vision is distorted.
- You may notice dark, blurry areas or white-out in the center of your vision.
- Color perception may be decreased or changed.

If you have any of these symptoms, see your ophthalmologist. Early treatment can save your vision!

FLAVONOIDS

Flavonoids, found in plants, are a diverse group of water-soluble pigments that benefit health. Flavonoids give plants their color. There are more than four thousand different flavonoids, offering protection from UV light and cardiovascular benefits. Flavonoids are widely distributed in plants and have many functions including producing yellow or red/blue pigmentation and protection from attack by microbes and insects. This group has been referred to as "nature's biological response modifiers" because of its ability to modify the body's reaction to allergens, viruses, and carcinogens. Many modern-day medicines are made from plant flavonoids. Older, less traditional medicines native to the United States contain flavonoids.

The flavonoids may be classified into six groups based on their structure.

THE CLASSES OF FLAVONOIDS

Flavonoid	Where to find it
Phenolic Acids	Found in red fruits, black radish, onions, and tea.
Flavonols	This is by far the best-represented category of flavonoid compounds. The flavonols are in almost everything that grows. They are present in highest concentration in onions, curly kale, leeks, broccoli, and blueberries. Red wine and tea have high amounts of flavonols. In fruit the flavonols accumulate in the skin and leaves, because sunlight stimulates their synthesis. Do you know that different concentrations exist between pieces of fruit on the same tree and even different sides of a piece of fruit? Within the plant, the flavonols are a sunscreen against UV damage. In leafy plants the darker outer leaves represent a higher flavonol concentration than the inner core.
Flavones	In contrast to the ubiquitous flavonols the flavones are relatively rare. Sources are parsley, celery, and the skin of citrus fruits.
Flavanones	The flavanones are in tomatoes and mint but the highest concentration is in citrus fruit. The white membranes separating orange segments have an extraordinarily high amount of

the flavanones. Eating a whole orange will give you five times as much as a glass of orange juice.[5]

Isoflavones

These are structurally similar to estrogen and are referred to as phytoestrogens because of their ability to bind to estrogen receptors. The main source of isoflavones is the soybean. Soy milk, tempeh, and miso are made from soybeans.

Flavonols

These flavonoids can be found in single forms, called catechins, or as multiples, called proanthocyanidins. Catechins are found in many fruits and red wine, but the highest concentrations are found in green tea and chocolate. When the catechins link together to form proanthocyanidins, they develop the ability to form complexes with salivary proteins, thus producing the astringent character of fruit (grapes, peaches, apples, pears, berries) and beverages (wines, ciders, teas, beers, etc.) and the bitterness of chocolate.

FLAVONOIDS IN TEAS

The flavonoid power molecules are of special interest with regard to teas.

Commercial teas, both green and black, are from the same plant, Camellia senensis. Camellia senensis leaves have high amounts of epigallo epicatechin, an EGCG. After the tea leaves are picked from the plant, the leaves begin to wilt. Wilting signifies that the chlorophyll in the leaves is decomposing and the flavonoids are becoming oxidized. In green tea processing, the oxidation process is stopped by heating the tea, leaving the green color and flavonoids intact. The processing of black tea allows the leaves to completely oxidize. The result of the different processing methods accounts for the higher concentration of flavonoids that remain in green tea. Because the flavonoids in tea are sensitive to changes in pH it has been speculated that they could be inactivated by milk in tea. This does not seem to be the case. Enjoy your tea with lemon or milk, as neither will affect the power molecules present.

The catechin flavonol, epigallocatechin-3-gallate (EGCG), is responsible for most of the protection offered by tea. The scope of presumed benefit is broad and includes protection against coronary heart disease, bacterial and viral infection, and even cancer. EGCG has also been shown to assist with weight reduction.

Tea has great benefits to the body. Brew your own real tea and do not think that the instant tea mixes or bottled teas are equivalent to the real thing. Because of the growing interest in the flavonoid content of food, the USDA performed an evaluation of commonly consumed foods, including teas. The USDA report confirmed the high-flavonoid content of green and black teas but showed instant green and black teas to be lacking in the power molecules.[6] The EGCG content of regular brewed green tea dropped from a high of 77mg/100g to only 3mg when the green tea was processed into the instant.

In Charleston, South Carolina, the Bigelow tea family has established the Charleston Tea Plantation. The plantation is open for tours and is a wonderful educational opportunity for anyone interested in tea. Each year newly picked Bigelow tea, called First Blush, is offered to visitors.

KEY FLAVONOIDS

- Quercetin has an anti-inflammatory effect by directly inhibiting the release of histamine and other allergic/inflammatory mediators. Histamine is released from the white blood cell early in the allergic response of seasonal allergies. Histamine causes the itching and watery eyes. Quercetin is found naturally in apples, green tea, and citrus fruit. Additionally, it is an antioxidant.
- Epicatechin aids blood flow, thereby improving cardiovascular health.

A functional food is a food that may provide a health benefit beyond the nutrients that it contains.[7] For example, tomatoes lower the risk of forming blood clots in addition to supplying vitamin C.[8]

Functional foods are an area of increasing interest to food companies. Unfortunately, the "function" of most of the newly created foods is to increase profits for the food companies. Sales of these foods topped $25 billion last year. Just because a product is labeled as having a benefit for the body doesn't necessarily mean it does. But rather than relying on artificial additives, I suggest focusing on the natural foods that will increase energy.

In 2000, the USDA published a list of the top antioxidant foods, demonstrating that the federal government saw benefit to adding these foods to our diets. In 2006, an expanded study of more than 1,100 foods was done.[9] Combined, both studies give us very good guidelines on where to find the most antioxidants in foods. But the later study went even further and speculated that the reason clinical trials evaluating the benefits of antioxidant supplements have not shown a benefit is because antioxidants do not occur in isolation. Rather, plants contain many different antioxidant compounds that cooperate in an integrated manner in plants, and may work together in our bodies. "Thus, a network of antioxidants with different chemical properties may be needed for proper protection against oxidative damage."[10] It is food itself that carries protection from oxidative damage, not a pill from the vitamin store. Studies have show that populations with the highest intake of antioxidant foods have a lower risk for cancer and heart disease.

"SHOULD I TAKE VITAMINS?"

My patients ask me this question every day. What I recommend is that you eat foods that naturally contain vitamins. Whole grains, vegetables, fruit, and nuts are optimal sources for vitamins and power molecules in natural occurring forms.

However, there are times when a vitamin supplement is warranted:

- Omega-3—If you do not eat fish, I recommend that you take an omega-3 fish oil capule—2000mg per day. Our diets are low in this important fat, so you must make a point of consuming oily fish or take a supplement. Consult *Consumer Reports* to make sure the one you are taking has what it should have. www.consumerreports.com
- Calcium—All females should take calcium citrate with vitamin D to prevent bone loss. I recommend 1500mg of calcium daily for all women older than fifty years and 1000mg for younger women.
- Vitamin D—There is an increased awareness of the necessity of consuming more vitamin D than was previously recommended. Vitamin D is necessary for calcium absorption and bone health. New research shows

that vitamin D assists the immune system, helping to prevent cancers from developing. It has been noted that people with high levels of vitamin D are at low risk for developing dementia. Our bodies make vitamin D naturally from sunlight. We know UV light from the sun raises the risk for skin cancer and premature aging of the skin. By avoiding the UV damage in sunlight, we deprive ourselves of vitamin D. Vitamin D is found in few foods, but milk is fortified with it. Food sources: 3½ ounces of salmon or mackerel have approximately 350 IU; IU is the abbreviation for International Units. Three ounces of canned tuna have 200 IU, 2 ounces of sardines have 250 IU, and 1 cup of fortified milk has 98 IU. I recommend that anyone over the age of forty, male or female, consume vitamin D_3 (the active form that our body can use)— 800 IU in supplement form. The average U.S. adult intake of vitamin D is only 230 IU daily. Many multivitamin formulations use the less potent vitamin D_2, instead of the more active D_3. We absorb vitamin D through our skin and digestive tract less efficiently as we age. I routinely measure vitamin D levels on new patients and I have found a high number of them are deficient in the vitamin. Suggest to your physician that he or she run a vitamin D level. If your levels are lower than 50ng/ml (nanogram per milliliter) you need to supplement this important mineral.

- Vitamin C—It is a good idea to take Vitamin C when your immune system is taxed or when you travel. Because it is a water-soluble vitamin, I recommend taking 500mg in the morning and in the evening. Start taking it before your air travel, continue during the trip, and for a day or so after you return.

TOP FIFTEEN ANTIOXIDANT FOODS

1.	Blackberries	9.	Blueberries
2.	Walnuts	10.	Ground cloves
3.	Strawberries	11.	Grape juice
4.	Artichokes	12.	Unsweetened chocolate
5.	Cranberries	13.	Cranberry juice
6.	Coffee	14.	Cherries
7.	Raspberries	15.	Red wine
8.	Pecans		

SOMETIMES YOU FEEL LIKE A NUT!

Nuts are a satisfying snack and can add pizzazz to vegetables and salads. The top three nuts: walnuts, pecans, and pistachios.

Walnuts—Walnuts appear on the USDA list because they contain the highest amount of omega-3 fat, a powerful anti-inflammatory agent.

Pecans—It might come as a surprise to you to see pecans on the list. But pecans have gotten a bad rap due to their association with pecan pie, delicious but high in sugar and fat. Pecans contain the minerals manganese, magnesium, and copper. Pecans are a great source of thiamin and vitamin B, important for our nerves. Pecans even contain EGCG, the antioxidant in green tea. Skip the pecan pie, though, because the high sugar will negate the nutritional advantage of this often overlooked source of power molecules.

Pistachios—Pistachios have vitamin B_6 and thiamin, and are high in the minerals potassium, phosphorous, magnesium, and manganese. Pistachios have vitamins E, A, B_6, and thiamin. If their green color made you suspect they contained the power molecules, you are right. Pistachios have a good amount of the flavonoid, catechin, which stimulates the immune system.

LIFE IS JUST A BOWL OF . . . CHERRIES!

Cherries have among the highest levels of antioxidants, containing about the same quantity as blueberries. A recent study conducted by University of Michigan researchers found that antioxidant-rich cherries helped reduce many of the risk factors for heart disease and metabolic syndrome by lowering total cholesterol levels, reducing triglycerides, lowering insulin and fasting glucose levels, lowering levels of a plasma marker of oxidative damage, increasing blood antioxidant capacity, and reducing "fatty liver." (www.choosecherries.com) Cherries are high in the flavonoid power molecules. They have benefits beyond basic nutrition. By virtue of their antioxidant properties they are "functional foods."

The fruit, vegetables, spices, and even the coffee that comes from nature are all functional foods from an antioxidant point of view. Antioxidants repair the damage from the wear and tear of living. Pomegranate is a powerhouse of antioxidants and has been shown to reduce systolic blood pressure and prevent the development of atherosclerosis. Walnuts are near the top of the list for good reason: Walnuts lower blood cholesterol and improve the ability for the coronary arteries to supply blood to the heart. In March 2004, the FDA accepted the following qualified health claim about walnuts: "Supportive but not conclusive research shows that eating 1.5 ounces per day of walnuts, as part of a low-saturated fat and low-cholesterol diet and not resulting in increased caloric intake may reduce the risk of coronary heart disease."

Blueberries, grape juice, and red wine are strong antioxidants in addition to containing resveratrol. Spices are also strong antioxidants and should be included in your diet. Spices listed in the top fifty antioxidants include cloves, oregano, ginger, cinnamon, turmeric, basil, mustard seed, parsley, and pepper.

GIVE A FIG

Fresh figs are delicious natural treats that are high in antioxidants and a good source of fiber. Figs are lusciously sweet with a chewy texture and crunchiness that comes from their seeds. They are also high in fiber, potassium, and manganese. California figs are available from June through September; some of the Mediterranean varieties are available through autumn. They make a perfect little pop-in-your-mouth snack or they can be tossed into salads.

Aim for nine servings of vegetables and fruit daily. I realize this may sound like a large amount, if you are not eating very many vegetables or fruits now. But keep in mind that a portion is one cup of uncooked vegetables or ½ cup cooked vegetables. To reach the magic number of nine servings it is essential to include a fruit and/or a vegetable with each meal. If you make a big salad your lunch of choice you are home free! A large salad easily contains three to four cups of leafy green vegetables; just add a serving of protein and you are all set.

EXAMPLE OF VEGETABLES AND FRUITS IN A TYPICAL DAY

Breakfast: One piece of fruit or ½ cup berries

Lunch: Salad of dark green leafy vegetables, combined with accents of red, yellow, and purple vegetables to equal four cups

Snack: One serving of fruit

Dinner: Two cooked vegetables

Dessert: One piece of fruit

Total for the day: Nine servings

PUMP UP YOUR RESVERATROL RESERVE

Resveratrol is a power molecule found in everyday foods we eat that gives protection to the heart and the body.

Resveratrol is a substance found in the skin of red grapes, blueberries, cranberries, and red-skinned peanuts. Scientists first became interested in resveratrol when its presence was detected in red wine; it was believed that it would help explain the "French paradox." In France, there is little cardiovascular disease despite a diet that is rich in high-fat cheese and cream. As a high-fat diet encourages the buildup of plaque in the arteries, scientists looked for an explanation to this conundrum (the French paradox). Research into the properties of resveratrol has shown it to be a powerful antioxidant that scavenges (neutralizes) free radicals and inhibits LDL oxidation (the buildup of harmful plaque).

FACTS ABOUT RESVERATROL

- Resveratrol stimulates the arteries to produce nitric oxide, allowing smooth muscle relaxation in arterial walls. When the arteries are relaxed blood flows more easily.

- Resveratrol inhibits platelet aggregation. During a heart attack platelets come together to form a clot. Resveratrol makes platelets "less sticky" so that they slide easily past one another, reducing the chance of forming a clot. Aspirin works in the same way.

- Resveratrol inhibits the proliferation of cancerous cells and signals apoptosis (cell death).

- Resveratrol is an inhibitor of inflammatory enzymes, including cyclooxygenase and lipoxygenase. The inflammatory cascade is part of a host of problems: atherosclerosis, arthritis, premature aging of the body. In fact, almost all chronic disease processes have an inflammatory component. Often elevation of the inflammation proteins is the first sign of a disease process, even before the patient notices any symptoms.

The benefits of resveratrol extend beyond the cardiovascular system and seem to reduce the tendency to develop inflammatory conditions and cancers. Recent discoveries showed that resveratrol has the ability to encourage the longevity gene, SIR1. When cells are exposed to a high amount of resveratrol, the longevity genes are turned on. It is like flipping on a light switch in a dark room.

VINEYARD VIGNETTES

When grapes ripen, sugars and flavonoids are formed. Flavonoids and resveratrol form as a reaction to the UV light hitting the grape. The riper the grape the more of these are found in the final wine. Resveratrol and flavonoids are found in the skin primarily; little is present within the flesh. Red wine, but not white wine, is fermented with the skins, allowing the wine to absorb resveratrol. Red wine contains higher amounts of resveratrol and flavonoids.

Wine is a complex liquid. Not only does it contain alcohol and water, its identity is recognizable because of the characteristic aromatic compounds (called terpenes, esters, and alcohols), sugars, and flavonoids (such as anthocyanins and tannins). The aroma of wine evolves as the by-products of fermentation, formed when sugar turns into alcohol. Other aroma compounds are formed during aging and result from oxidation. The subtle development of aroma and taste is one of wine's intriguing aspects.

Tannins are flavonoids found in the skin of fruit and grapes that interact strongly with proteins. This interactive property is the fundamental role of tannins. Tannins interact with the salivary proteins. When you eat a piece of unripened fruit it is sensed as being astringent and sharp. Because ripening changes the composition of the tannins, the ripe fruit has a sweet taste. Tannins are also antioxidants and protect the wine from oxidation. Theoretically wine that is meant to be aged contains high amounts of tannins. As wine ages tannins are masked by products of fermentation. It is the combination of the fermented wine with the tannins that gives a well-aged wine complexity and unique taste.

GOOD NEWS FOR CHOCOHOLICS

Many recent studies have touted the health benefits of red wine and tea, as they are high in antioxidants. Cocoa is also rich in these compounds. If you want to avoid extra calories, stay away from the sugar and high-fat content dairy products that are common additives to cocoa. Substitute nonfat milk and use Splenda to sweeten the cocoa.

Although you can enjoy cocoa either hot or cold, the hot version tends to trigger the release of more antioxidants than its cold counterpart. A normal 40g bar of chocolate contains about 8g of saturated fat, compared to only 0.3g in an average cup of hot cocoa.

THE BENEFITS OF CACAO

Chocolate is high in flavonoids and antioxidants, and contains theobromo-cocoa, a substance that acts in the brain in a similar way to opioids. Dark chocolate contains the flavonoids epicatechin and garlic acid, which may lower blood pressure. Dark chocolate has actually been shown to lower cholesterol, too.

All chocolate is made from cacao beans. They contain no sugar and between 12 and 50 percent fat, depending on the variety and growing conditions. Cacao is remarkably rich in magnesium, which is cited as the primary reason most women crave chocolate during their menstrual period. Cacao nibs are pieces of raw chocolate, and they are a real treat.

GUILTLESS CHOCOLATE

Not exactly, but these are healthier versions of the sweet stuff you may be craving.

- Green & Black's Organic Dark Chocolate—Yummy smooth dark bittersweet chocolate. www.greenandblacksdirect.com
- Scharffen Berger Chocolate Covered Roasted Cacao Nibs— Semisweet coated cacao nibs. www.artisanconfection.com

NEED AN INSTANT ENERGY BOOST?

Food sources of the power molecule resveratrol are red and purple grapes, blueberries, and red-skinned peanuts. They should be a "go-to" snack when you need a little something for an energy boost. Blueberries and red grapes containing resveratrol are carbohydrates; combine them with a protein like yogurt or low-fat cottage cheese to ensure a continuous energy supply.

RESVERATROL QUICK PICK-ME-UPS

- ½ cup blueberries and wheat germ with Fage Total yogurt—use either 2 percent or 0 percent fat varieties or try Stonyfield Farm Fat-Free Organic yogurt.
- A glass of cabernet with 2 ounces of low-fat Gouda or Jarlsberg Light.

DRINK TO YOUR HEALTH

Beer is made from hops, a form of grain, and fermented, producing alcohol. It contains a small amount of the flavonol catechin. Red wine contains more catechins, other flavonoid forms, and resveratrol. From a nutritional perspective, red wine has more benefit to the body than beer. The recommended amount is one glass for a female and two glasses for a male. But don't overdo it, and be conscious of the fact that alcohol consumption can escalate over time if you are not careful.

CHAPTER SEVEN

OMEGA-3: KING OF LAND AND SEA

Nature does nothing uselessly.

—ARISTOTLE

You must consume fat if you want to be healthy and energetic. You cannot live without fat. Essential fatty acids are fats that our bodies cannot make and we must consume. We need them to make cell membranes, hormones, neurotransmitters, and cellular components. Essential fats allow us to remember, keep our hearts beating, and allow us to develop sexually; in short, they influence every aspect of life. There are two types of essential fatty acids, omega-6 and omega-3. (In chemistry terms, the name refers to the location of the first double bond. In the omega-6 fats, the first double bond is after the sixth carbon; in the omega-3 fats, it is after the third carbon.) We require both omega-3 and omega-6 fats to be in top health.

The biggest problem with the typical Western diet is that it contains far more omega-6 than omega-3. Both fats come from plants. Plants store omega-6 fat as linoleic acid (the proper chemical name) within the seeds. Omega-3 fat (linolenic) is formed when the seed germinates. The relationship between the two fats is important. Omega-6 is the storage form of energy, while omega-3 is the active form of energy in young plants.

NATURE OR MAGIC TRICK?

Omega-3 in a plant actually captures the energy of sunlight and changes it into starch. The plant's ability to grow depends on omega-3 fat. Without omega-3 fat, our life on earth would not exist. When I was a biology student, I was astounded to learn that plants have specialized organs, called chloroplasts, that harvest light and transform it into physical matter. Photosynthesis transforms light into actual components of plants. It sounded like magic to me! The omega-3 fat in the chloroplast membrane (thylacoid membrane) enables the transformation of photons into plant leaves.

The oceans and rivers are a source of one of the most health-promoting substances on earth: omega-3 fats in the bodies of fish. While the major source of protein in the Western diet has been meat, studies in the last twenty years have increasingly suggested that high amounts of grain-fed meat are poor choices nutritionally.

Two factors cause the ill health associations:

1. The volume of meat eaten is so much greater than the amount of fish. Each American consumes 195 pounds of meat per year, more than twice the 57 pounds that was consumed in 1950. Fish consumption is slightly more than 35 pounds per person per year.

2. The way meat is raised promotes unnaturally fat animals. Animals raised for consumption are fed grain, rather than allowing them to graze. Because the animals eat so much grain, containing omega-6 fat, their body fat is composed of omega-6 fat and saturated fat. The cows will gain weight more rapidly on this diet. (If animals are allowed to graze, their fat contains both omega-6 and omega-3.) By the way, the same works for humans: if our diets are high in omega-6 fat our body fat will have high amounts of omega-6 fat. If our diets have high amounts of grain we will easily gain weight.

All living things have fat: plants, animals, fish, and humans. Fat is vital for building membranes and synthesizing hormones. Protein and fat are always found together. But all fat is not the same. Saturated fat, from grain-fed animals, raises cholesterol, both total cholesterol and the harmful LDL cholesterol. High saturated fat in the diet is associated with atherosclerosis and coronary artery disease. Dean Ornish, M.D., the eminent cardiologist, recommends eliminating saturated fat from our diet entirely and relying only on plants and fish to satisfy our protein requirements.

EAT MORE FISH; EAT LESS MEAT

My approach is somewhat different. I suggest that you increase the amount of omega-3 in your diet by consuming more fish and leafy greens while cutting back on the saturated fat. Eat more fish; eat less meat. The high amounts of saturated fat in our diets predispose our organs to oxidative stress and inflammation. When you do eat meat, eat meat that is naturally raised by grazing. Besides saturated fat, we need to limit the amount of omega-6 fat.

The sources of omega-3 depend on the animal's diet. Fish have the most omega-3 because they only eat omega-3 foods. Therefore anything that lives in the sea contains omega-3 fat, including shrimp, clams, and other shellfish. Oily fish (such as tuna, wild salmon, sardines, halibut, herring, cod, catfish, and mackerel) have more.

The fat contained in fish has proven health benefits that were first noted in the Inuit people by Hans Olaf Bang and Jørn Dyerberg, scientists from Denmark. They noticed that although the Inuits of Greenland had an exceptionally high-fat diet, they had virtually no heart disease. At the time it was thought that high-fat diets led to heart attacks and other cardiovascular disease. Bang and Dyerberg traveled to Greenland to evaluate the Inuit diet and to obtain blood samples of the residents. They discovered that it was indeed high in fat (about 50 percent) and the fat was from the bodies of seals and fish. Blubber was a staple of the diet. The blood samples revealed low levels of triglycerides and LDL (bad) cholesterol and high HDL (good) cholesterol—a cholesterol profile known to offer protection against cardiovascular disease. Bang and Dyerberg had hit upon a nutritional milestone—the fat in fish protects the heart.

In 2001, an Italian study confirmed the importance of fats from fish for the heart. This landmark study, the GISSI study, followed eleven thousand Italian men who had recovered from heart attacks. Half of the men were given fish-oil capsules and the other half were given vitamin E capsules. After one year there was a 45 percent decrease in cardiac death in the group that took the fish-oil capsules. The interesting fact about the GISSI study is that it showed benefit to the heart even in a group that was known to have heart disease. Today in Italy fish-oil capsules are the standard care after a heart attack.[1]

Earlier this year a Japanese study was published tracking eighteen thousand people who regularly ate fish but who had high cholesterol. They were given either fish-oil capsules with a drug to reduce cholesterol or just a drug to reduce cholesterol and followed for five years. This study again confirmed the protective value of fish oil on the heart with a lower number of major cardiac events in the group who consumed fish oil.[2] Fat from fish is anti-inflammatory.

HOW OMEGA-3 FATS WORK

Omega-3 fats act to thin the blood naturally. They keep the lining of the arteries smooth, clear of thickening and inflammation. They act as a natural anticoagulant by altering the ability of platelets in your blood to clump together.

Research has suggested that a diet rich in omega-3 fats can:

- Reduce the risk of cardiovascular disease.
- Decrease risk of irregular heart rhythms (arrhythmias), which can lead to sudden cardiac death.
- Decrease levels of triglycerides—a type of fat found in the blood which has been linked to heart disease.
- Reduce the clumping of small particles in the blood called platelets, which can cause potentially harmful clots.
- Decrease growth rate of the fatty plaques that can clog up the arteries.
- Lower blood pressure.

Research has suggested that omega-3 fats can cut the risk of cancers such as prostate and skin. Other work has suggested that a diet rich in omega-3 can help improve behavior in violent and antisocial teenagers. They have also been touted as a treatment for asthma and inflammatory-bowel disease. Studies are currently under way to test the possibility that the omega-3 fats could even prevent memory loss and dementia.

What About the Fat in Plants?

All green leafy plants have omega-3 fat. Grains have omega-6 fat. Commercially raised beef cattle have little omega-3 in their bodies because their grain diets simply do not supply it. By allowing animals to graze they accumulate omega-3 fat within their bodies. Free-range animals have a mixture of omega-6 and omega-3 fats in their bodies, as a result. Fish eat algae, plankton, and other fish; all are sources of omega-3 fat. Fish are composed only of omega-3 fats because of their diet.

Green plants would seem to be the "all-purpose" nutrient in that they help us to feel full, supply vitamins and minerals, and contain power molecules and healthy omega-3 fat. Europeans eat green plants in greater quantities than Americans. Greeks and Italians have dozens of leafy vegetables that Americans are unfamiliar with. If you ever have the chance, I suggest visiting an open-air market in Europe to witness firsthand the beautifully displayed, freshly picked produce.

Turn Over a New Leaf

To add more variety to your meals, venture into unknown territory with some of the following leafy green vegetables. The green leafy vegetables listed contain omega-3 fat as well as a multitude of antioxidants, power molecules, and vitamins. Experiment—it's the best way to find new favorites.

All of these have benefits to your health:

- **Arugula.** Arugula is also called rocket or roquette or Italian cress. Arugula is frequently used in salads. There are many varieties, with the larger leafed types being quite bitter. Everyone likes the baby-leaf type as a salad green; so if arugula is unfamiliar, you may want to add baby leaves in your usual salad mix. If you are a gardener, try growing arugula because it is frost resistant and grows rapidly. (Maybe that is why it is called rocket!)

- **Chicory.** Chicory comes in a variety of colors from green to red. Chicory has a tart taste and is best used as an accent to milder salad greens. Cooked briefly, just enough to soften the leaves, it turns into a tasty side dish.
- **Collard Greens.** Collards will remind me always of my very young childhood when I visited my grandmother. My grandmother grew these on her farm and served them with black-eyed peas. Unlike the Southern tradition of boiling collard greens, she would just steam them lightly and top them with melted butter. I make them just the same way but I substitute olive oil.
- **Dandelions.** As I write this I am reminded of a patient, a Greek woman of eighty, who loves dandelions and orders them several times a week from Grace's Marketplace in New York City. She related how she learned to cook dandelions in Greece and was so delighted with my approval that she brought me a present of the dandelions that she had graciously prepared. They were just delicious, boiled and tossed with olive oil and a small amount of garlic. They contain vitamins A, C, and K. Dandelions are also a source of lutein and zeaxanthin for vision. (Please do not pick the dandelions from your lawn—especially if it has been sprayed with chemicals or fertilizers.)
- **Kale.** Kale is a highly nutritious vegetable from the cabbage family. Discard the thick stems, steam, and toss with olive oil and lemon. Kale contains high amounts of vitamins K and A and omega-3.
- **Mustard Greens.** Mustard greens are delicious and packed with nutrition, containing good amounts of plant protein and omega-3 fat. They are a concentrated source of vitamins C, A, K, and folate. Mustard greens should be on the list of foods that pregnant women are advised to consume. In addition to vitamins, mustard greens supply lutein and zeaxanthin for vision.
- **Purslane.** When I lecture about omega-3 I always ask, "Who in the audience has heard of purslane?" It is rare for anyone to answer in the affirmative. This plant is packed with power molecules and I really hope we will see it used more in the States. I first heard of purslane through the work of Artemis Simopoulos, M.D., a Greek American who has written extensively on the importance of omega-3 fat in the diet. Dr. Simopoulos documented that purslane contains more omega-3

fat than any known leafy plant. Native to the arid hills of Greece, thought to be a weed by many, purslane has an omega-3 content four times that of cultivated spinach. By all means, add purslane to your salads; you will enjoy its delicate flavor and texture. Good luck finding it in your local store; you might enjoy growing your own as it is very hardy.

- **Swiss Chard.** There are three varieties: red, green, and rainbow. Swiss chard is a member of the beet family and contains vitamins A, C, and K. It is delicious in salads or can be cooked and served as a side dish. Try my recipe for a Swiss Chard and Ricotta Omelet (page 176).

Vegetables containing the fat-soluble vitamins—vitamins D, E, A, and K—should be consumed with a sprinkling of oil to help your body absorb them. I suggest you use olive oil, walnut oil, or canola oil. These oils will benefit your health. Avoid any vegetable oil such as peanut, corn, or soybean oil; they are omega-6 oils and we have enough of those in our diets. Olive oil is monounsaturated oil. Walnut and canola oils have omega-3 fat.

SAMPLE OMEGA-3 QUICK PICK-ME-UP

- A handful of walnuts are satisfying and have nine times more omega-3 fat than any other nut.
- A hard-boiled omega-3 egg has 8g protein and 150mg omega-3 fat. Don't worry about the cholesterol in that egg—the omega-3 fat cancels it out!
- Lunch on the run could be a pop-top 3-ounce can of dark Italian tuna packed in olive oil (drain well) with a Ziploc bag of raw vegetables.

Don't follow the old wives' tale of taking cod liver oil to stay healthy. The liver contains high amounts of vitamin A. This is not a good source of omega-3.

BE AN OMEGA-3 DETECTIVE

Omega-3 fats have enormous benefits for us. Learn to search for new ways of consuming them! The omega-3 fats from the bodies of fish are: eicosapentaenoic acid (EPA) and docosahexaenoic acid (DHA). The plant form of omega-3 fat is alpha linoleic acid (ALA). Making healthy, energizing food choices just got easier thanks to an expanding crop of omega-3 products in the dairy case—milk, yogurt, eggs, and cheese. Switch from regular low- or nonfat dairy products to delicious, satisfying omega-3 enriched dairy products.

Per gram, the foods highest in the omega-3 fatty acid DHA include: caviar, salmon, mackerel, shad, anchovies, whitefish, steelhead trout, herring, tuna, sardines, Rainbow trout.[3]

OMEGA 3 HEROES

Walnut oil—400mg per 1-ounce serving

Walnuts—190mg per 1-ounce serving

Flaxseed Oil—2000mg per 1-ounce serving

Omega-3 Enriched Egg—150–350mg per egg

Caviar—1000mg per 2-ounce serving

Salmon—1000mg per 3-ounce serving

Shrimp—700mg per 5-ounce serving

The quantity of omega-3 depends on the animal's diet. Fish have the most omega-3 because they eat only omega-3 foods.

GENES AND FAT

Because fat is so important to our bodies it should not come as a surprise that fat has an effect on our genes, allowing the genes to code for proteins.[4] Studies have shown that high amounts of omega-6 fats cause the genes to produce a cancer-inducing protein, ras p21. But high amounts of omega-3 fat silence the gene.[5] Both colon and breast cancers appear to be affected by the ras signal. This finding would explain the mechanism whereby populations consuming high amounts of omega-3 fat are protected from cancers of the breast and colon. The power molecule, omega-3, silences the death gene, ras p21, and promotes the longevity genes!

INFLAMMATION

Inflammation is a trigger to the development of atherosclerosis and various autoimmune diseases. The body requires a balance of inflammatory and anti-inflammatory fats. Fats that promote inflammation are omega-6 fats; we need them to fight off infection. Anti-inflammatory fats—omega-3 fats—keep the proteins produced by the inflammation response from getting out of hand.

TRADE YOUR CHARDONNAY FOR A CABERNET!

Wine consumption should not be more than two glasses per day for a man, and no more than one glass for a woman at four ounces per glass—red wine preferably.

ANTIOXIDANT ENERGY COCKTAILS—THESE ARE A GREAT WAY TO DRINK YOUR ANTIOXIDANTS!

- *Ginger Juice Sparkler*—The ginger juice may be purchased at Whole Foods or online at www.gingerpeople.com. For a refreshing twist, use one teaspoon ginger juice in a glass of sparkling water with ice, and add a slice of orange or a sprig of mint.

- *Green Tea Citrus Cooler*—Make a mixture of equal parts limeade and lemonade, sweeten with a small amount of agave nectar or a small amount of sugar. Then add two cups brewed green tea. Serve in a pitcher with raspberries as a garnish.

- *Sun Tea*—Take whatever tea you like and put two to three teabags (either green or black tea) per quart of water depending on desired strength into a clear glass jar. Place jar in direct sunlight for a minimum of 3 hours. The longer it steeps in the sun, the stronger the flavor. Then refrigerate or serve over ice. It is optional to add sugar, agave nectar, or Splenda, fresh fruit slices, and mint into the jar *after* it steeps for added flavor.

CHAPTER EIGHT

THE ENERGY WORKOUT

People don't die of old age, they die of inactivity.

—*Jack La Lanne*

We know that exercise benefits the body. The benefit of aerobic exercise at every age is overwhelming: It decreases the risk of death. Even for the very old, exercise offers protection against dying. Daily exercise is a must.

Aerobic exercise also increases your energy level. Aerobic exercise means breathing hard and sweating. Because your muscles are working harder they require more oxygen—that explains the breathing. Sweating is your body's natural cooling mechanism. All body proteins are heat sensitive, meaning temperature changes their shape and we need to keep the body core within a narrow range of just a few degrees. That's why when the weather is cold we shiver—to raise core temperature. Likewise, when our muscles contract (producing heat) we sweat to cool our core. These mechanisms protect body proteins. But if you stress the muscles consistently with aerobic exercise, the muscles synthesize new capillaries to meet the demand. They also create more mitochondria, the cellular energy factories. Muscles also increase their production of enzymes as they become stronger. The heart and lungs become more efficient. The pumping strength of the heart is increased by aerobic exercise. Over time the exercise that you once found challenging is easy. In fact, any activity seems easier because you have become aerobically fit. Not only has exercise made the muscles stronger, it has strengthened the entire body with new capillaries and a more efficient circulatory system. You have more energy.

Aerobic exercise is the crucial part of the equation for most people. Be consistent with your exercise. Muscles respond to regular stimulation for capillaries, mitochondria, and enzymes to be made. It is tough to get going but you will be rewarded by renewed energy. Take a clue from Nike, Inc., "Just do it!"

> You burn ten times the number of calories by walking up stairs than by walking on a flat surface, and 4.5 times as many walking down stairs.

FINDING A GOOD TRAINER

A great certified trainer can make the difference between working out and not making any progress. In achieving results, having an expert to guide you step-by-step may seem like a luxury, but it can be a worthwhile investment in your health and well-being. Most of us need some coaching, mentoring, and training that working with an expert offers.

But just because he or she has the physique of an Olympic medalist doesn't mean he knows anything about fitness and physiology or that he has mastered the art of motivation. You will want to avoid spending a fortune on someone who received his training online or by mail. For example, certified trainers may have areas of specialization such as weight management, weight training, and strength training.

Here are some simple steps to take to ensure that you have done your homework before you sign up.

I.   Be sure to check out the credentials of any fitness expert you are considering. Experts come with varying degrees of expertise, and many are certified in more than one area of specialization. Ask what kind of education and training they received and which certifications and licenses they hold, and what their particular field of interest is. The top certifications are by the American College of Sports Medicine (ACSM), the National Strength and Conditioning Association (NSCA), and the National Academy of Sports Medicine (NASM). Ask for references.

2.   What is the policy regarding cancellation? It is best to establish this in advance. Today most trainers require twenty-four-hour cancellation. Make sure they carry liability insurance. They should request a health screening from your doctor before starting you on an exercise program if you have not exercised in a long time.

3.   Set up a regular time and stick with it. This will establish a routine. If you are coming down with a cold or do not feel well, I suggest that you keep your appointment. Sure, you won't have your normal intensity but at least you can do a light workout. For years, this has been my policy and it has never, not once, made me feel worse. Of course, if you are really sick or have a fever—by all means, cancel.

4.   Get yourself a new trainer if you are wasting time talking. The trainer is not there to be your new best friend and you are not there to advise him about his personal life. If you are fortunate enough to have a trainer, then work it. And move your body and not your mouth.

SQUEEZING FITNESS INTO YOUR LIFE

In today's fast-paced world, finding time for fitness can be difficult. The key to making exercise part of your busy day is to make it convenient and keep it fun. Physical exercise is a prerequisite for energy.

With 1,440 minutes in each day, it shouldn't be that hard to find one hour a day for exercise. But it can be. For many people, days are a blur of work, household chores, errands, time with family and friends, and, of course, sleep. With everything going on, finding the time for exercise can be a challenge.

Still, even my patients who have the busiest schedules manage to find time for fitness. The key is to make it as convenient as possible for your particular lifestyle.

SNEAK IN SOME EXERCISE

Wake up early. Try getting up thirty minutes earlier than you normally do and use the extra time to walk on your treadmill or take a brisk walk around the neighborhood. Research suggests that people who exercise in the morning are more likely than are others to stick with it over the long term.

Do housework. Mop the floor, scrub the bathtub, or do other housework. The stretching and lifting are good exercise. Work at a fast pace to get your heart pumping. Put on some music.

Mow the lawn. Prune your trees, plant your flower bed, or mow the lawn. Gardening can burn up to three hundred calories an hour and is a great way to build strength. Raking and hoeing strengthen your arms and back, and digging works your arm and leg muscles.

End your day with a walk after work. Want to unwind after a stressful day? Walk off your stress. Bypass the taxi, subway, or bus and throw on a pair of comfortable shoes (or change into your Nikes or Reeboks) and power walk your way home or back from the train station, or just take a stroll. Exercising before dinner may also suppress your appetite, helping to reduce your total daily calorie intake.

Get your dog into the act. Take two quick walks with Fido or Fluffy every day. It's best to build up to about thirty minutes of continuous activity. But two fifteen-minute jaunts are nearly as good.

Exercise while watching TV. Use hand weights, ride a stationary bike, or do a stretching routine. Get up off the couch to change the channel on the TV. Or keep the telephone in another room so that you have to walk to answer it.

Henry, one of my patients, keeps his stability ball in his study and does crunches while watching TV; just this small change has enabled him to do one hundred extra crunches nightly.

Make family time exercise time. Take group walks after dinner or schedule a family game of kickball for Saturday mornings. Wait about an hour after you eat before exercising, however. Family excursions like hiking, skiing, canoeing, sailing, or exploring are wonderful. Your children will love it and by seeing the value you give to physical exercise, they will incorporate exercise into their own lives. You do not have to be a super athlete, you are already a superhero in their eyes. Children remember these excursions. My son, Matthew, to this day says his favorite family vacation was the one spent rafting on the Salmon River in Utah!

June is a forty-one-year-old teacher and mother of three daughters, age two, age three, and a newborn, who visited my office after the birth of her last child. Her weight had steadily increased after the birth of each child until her weight was 218 pounds. June is tall (five foot ten) with a large frame, so she can afford to carry a few extra pounds but she was clearly too heavy. Her cholesterol profile was fine and she was in good health so far. She was concerned about her family history of obesity; her mother and her sister were obese. June was constantly tired and felt she was headed in the wrong way healthwise. With a job and three small children, this working mother had little time to herself but realized the necessity of getting her life under control. I gave her a plan of healthy food and one Everyday Nutrition shake per day, and the weight began to roll off. I insisted that she begin an exercise program that would include daily aerobic exercise. June lived in SoHo near the Hudson River; she made a plan of daily morning walks along the water. In the beginning this was very challenging for her. But with time, as she became more fit, the walks increased and she was able to include arm exercise with the Power Belt. (The Power Belt is fastened around the waist and has cords with tension, which give resistance as the arms are pumped while walking. It not only firms the arms but is an effective way to elevate the heart rate while exercising.) What worked for June can work for anyone. Include protein in all meals, exercise every day, and eliminate processed foods. June has lost weight and gained more energy. She is radiant, exercises daily, cooks beautifully for her family, and is continuing to lose weight. Because of her family history, keeping her weight down will always be a challenge, but June has all the tools and is doing everything right, as of now. So if you really want it, you can make it happen. Teach your children how to achieve good health by practicing it yourself. June is a beautiful role model for her daughters.

MAKE IT AN ESCAPE

Enjoy your privacy. Some people enjoy the privacy of exercising at home and can work it into their home life fairly easily. For others, being at home may be too much of a distraction.

Be social. You may enjoy exercise as a social activity and do better with the encouragement of others. Look into dance clubs, hiking groups, health clubs, and tennis clubs. My husband and I are learning the tango.

Join a team. Try the softball, soccer, or volleyball team at your company or through your local parks and recreation department. Making a commitment to a team is a great motivator.

Join a fitness club near your office. Sign up for a spinning class that meets right before or after work, or during your lunch hour.

A walk in the park. Enjoy family time, but stay active. Doing it together makes it more fun. Take a hike in a local park, or bring your family to the beach to play a robust game of softball.

Run your errands. When you go to the mall or grocery store, park all the way at the end of the parking lot and walk the extra distance. It's a good idea to keep a pair of walking shoes in the trunk of your car so you're always ready when you have an extra half hour to do some exercise.

KEEP IT FUN!

Gloria first visited my office two years ago. She had elevated cholesterol and had gained twenty pounds. She worked long hours as an architect. Because of her schedule she reasoned that she did not have time for exercise and, she reasoned, she was too tired to exercise. I explained that exercise was a "nonnegotiable." So Gloria agreed to sign on with a personal trainer and start an exercise program. By having an appointment, she was committed to doing it. And to her surprise, she enjoyed exercising. One day she heard Lance Armstrong announce that the upcoming Tour de France was to be his last race. She turned to her husband to say that it would be a phenomenal idea to fly to France and witness the event. Her husband suggested that

they would be better able to view the event, without the hassle of fly-
ing, on television. Gloria did not agree, and decided to go to France
by herself. She made her own reservations in a small chic Parisian
hotel (her husband had always insisted on staying at the Ritz) and
enjoyed the wonderful museums of Paris on her own prior to the
race. When the great day arrived, she was among the crowds waving
the American flag at the Arc de Triomphe. The time came when the
cyclists approached the arch in the distance; closer and closer they
came, eventually circling it. But she could not see Lance! As they cir-
cled three times, she was able to see him. The strong and motivated
cyclist, her hero, the great Lance Armstrong—the reason she had
come to France. But the truth was she had come to Paris because of
her zest for life and desire to experience the moment. Gloria's story
does not stop here. On the plane home she read in a magazine that
Lance Armstrong was hosting a cross-country ride benefiting children with cancer. Gloria resolved to ride the last twenty miles of the
race. There was only one small problem: she had not been on a bicycle since she was seven years old! So, I found her a trainer who taught
her how to ride in Central Park and she worked until she was com-
petent riding in a group of cyclists. She fell a few times, but Gloria
persevered until she mastered the bicycle, flew to Texas, and rode
with Lance! The moral of Gloria's story is that you can have more
fun than you can imagine if you are willing to take some chances.

WORKOUT AT WORK

Make the most of your commuting time. Walk to work. Some of my patients ride
their bikes to their office. If you ride the bus to and from work, get off a few
blocks early and walk the rest of the way.

Take the stairs whenever you can. If you have a meeting on the fourteenth floor,
get off the elevator a few floors early and use the stairs.

Take fitness breaks instead of coffee breaks. Spend the time taking a fifteen-minute walk.

Start a lunchtime walking group with your coworkers. The regular routine and the
support of your coworkers may help you stick with the program.

Schedule exercise as you would any other appointment. Don't change your exercise plans if something else comes along—remind yourself that exercise is just as important.

When you travel, pack and plan so that you can stick to an exercise routine. Bring your jump rope or choose a hotel that has fitness facilities. If you're stuck in an airport waiting for a plane, grab your carry-on and take a walk.

Robert is an investment banker in his forties, born in Europe. He came to see me when he noticed that he was running out of steam. He has a passion for chocolate stemming from his childhood in Switzerland, and tends to nibble on chocolate in the afternoon. He never eats breakfast, and often has a bowl of pasta at business lunches, which was making him tired in the afternoon. Although he lives just down the block from a great gym which he belongs to, Robert historically has a hard time forcing himself to go work out. Something always got in the way. I suggested to him that since he spent more time in his office than he did in his co-op apartment on the Upper West Side, he should find a gym in midtown to go to right after he left the office, no matter what time that was. That was the plan for Robert: He would start his day with an Everyday Nutrition shake to get his protein, skip the heavy gnocchi or fettuccini at lunchtime, and do a daily workout, even if it was only fifteen minutes on the treadmill. We hit the jackpot for Robert. He stuck to his plan and in six weeks, his waist went down by a full notch in his Gucci belt, and he felt so terrific that even his girlfriend noticed his newfound stamina and called to thank me.

The moral of this story is let your individual lifestyle, job, and family responsibilities be your guide as to what is the best time and place for you to get your exercise. You have to do what works for you. Whatever option you choose, make daily exercise a habit you keep, and keep it fun, too!

BEFORE WORKING OUT

Drink a big glass of water. If you enjoy coffee, that is okay, too. Contrary to popular belief, caffeine is not dehydrating. But be aware that caffeine is a bladder irritant. By drinking it your workout will be interrupted by a bathroom break. I recommend water to my patients.

AFTER WORKING OUT

Have a protein snack after exercising. Exercise causes minute tears in muscle fiber; it is through repairing the tears that muscle becomes stronger. Only protein can repair the minute tears. New studies show that if protein is consumed right after a workout, muscle strength is improved. Because my Everyday Nutrition shakes contain 20g high-quality protein they are ideal for a postexercise snack.

NOT ALL EXERCISE IS CREATED EQUAL!

Our bodies have two separate aerobic systems. One system allows us to perform long-duration activity, while the other system is focused toward intense hunting-like activity.

The slow system works when we go on long walks or do easy work, like gardening. The muscles use fat for fuel during slow aerobic activity. This, of course, is good news. Many people might think that they aren't doing anything for their bodies but in fact, the slow aerobic exercise means endurance. Endurance benefits the lungs, heart, muscles, and mind—there is not one bodily system that doesn't derive benefit from slow aerobic activity. This is the metabolic pace where your body grows and adapts to exercise. Indeed the reason the body stores fat in the first place is just so it will be available. Fat stores are broken down to supply energy during long-duration activity. We feel great, refreshed, and elated after our slow aerobic exercise.

The second system, or fast system, is engaged when we take exercise to the next level. For example, on a leisurely aerobic walk when we begin to run we move from a slow fat-burning system to the fast system. At this pace we require a different fuel source; we require more power than is supplied by breaking down fat alone so the muscles use glucose. From an evolutionary perspective, we ran from danger and hunted with this system activated. Watch a wild animal stalk its prey: their pupils dilate, their attention is entirely focused, and they then spring into action running at top speed to conquer their prey. On this level the animal's muscles cannot work any harder. It is the fast system that ensures survival.

How do we know when the fast system is activated? Our heart rate will tell us. To supply more oxygen to the rapidly exercising muscles, the heart beats faster. It is at 70 percent of the peak heart rate that the fast system is kicked into gear. Over 70 percent of the peak heart rate and you have moved into a different metabolism! We need both systems for top energy. Slow aerobic exercise builds endurance and prevents decline. Fast aerobic exercise enables us to achieve our peak activity. Activities that bring you into the fast aerobic zone are those where you are really pushing yourself close to your maximal capability. Think of it this way: If you were being chased by a tiger, you would not walk briskly or jog. You would run!

Alan, age forty, is a former professional rugby player turned banker. He has been highly athletic his entire life. It seemed fitting that when Alan married he would chose Natalie, herself a track star throughout her college and high school years. Weekends are spent together playing golf or tennis or with friends tossing the football in Central Park. Last year Alan thought it might be fun to enter his firm's annual sprint, held on Memorial Day. For the past five years the race had been dominated by a man who ran track in college. To the competitive Alan, this sounded like the perfect challenge—he would take the title away from the current champ. Only one problem: Alan had never run in a race before! Well, he was in great shape, however, and, in his prime, had been considered the star player of his rugby team. And don't forget Alan is married to Natalie, a former track star; the logical solution was to ask Natalie to give him a few pointers. So one fine spring day Alan and Natalie suited up in their gym attire and headed off to Central Park to analyze Alan's running skills. Natalie soon realized that Alan would require serious training to make a respectable showing and, hopefully, win. Alan had tremendous endurance but lacked the burst of power that running a short race requires. Alan could easily run for long distances. But he did not run fast. This was not good news for someone who wanted to win a sprint! Although Alan was a strong athlete, he had emphasized the slow aerobic training and neglected to train the fast aerobic system. With the race two months away, Alan began a serious training program of wind sprints. Supervised by Natalie, Alan's time became faster. He was activating his fast aerobic system and training his muscles to help him surge forward. It was fun and encouraging for him to see his time improve. But would it be good enough to win? On the day of the race Alan did just that. He won. Alan won because he had preferentially trained his fast aerobic system. He took his exercise to a new level.

Just as the already fit Alan had neglected his fast aerobic system, so do almost 100 percent of the people who come into my office. I hate to break this to you, but Pilates or yoga or brisk walking do not touch the fast aerobic system. To train in the zone of fast aerobics you need to be breathing very hard and sweating. You do not need to stay in the fast aerobic zone for a long time, but you do need to get there. The benefits of training in the fast aerobic zone are that you will move up your fitness level. And everything becomes easier. It is almost as if you magically become ten years younger!

OUR MUSCLE FIBERS

Our muscles are composed of two types of fibers: fast-twitch and slow-twitch fibers. The slow-twitch muscle fibers are responsible for sustained endurance exercise. Marathon runners have plenty of slow-twitch fibers. During a marathon the slow-twitch leg muscles contract tirelessly over hours of running. Fast-twitch fibers are the power generators for muscles. Fast-twitch fibers give a fast burst of speed. Baseball pitchers use fast-twitch muscle fibers when they throw a ball. Basketball players and gymnasts use fast-twitch fibers when they jump. All muscles have both types of fibers.

It is important to include training of the fast fibers because studies have shown that as we age the fast fibers numbers decrease. That means the power necessary to run after a bus or from a mugger or the power to do the salsa or get to the drop shot is gone. But the loss is preventable and reversible if you train the fast fibers. So include training in the fast aerobic zone.

FAST AEROBIC MOVES

- Intervals
- Jumping rope
- Wind sprints
- Throwing the medicine ball with force

When you work at the fast aerobic level you synthesize new capillaries to feed the muscles; the heart and lungs work at a higher level, and the fast-twitch muscle fibers are recruited. Fast-twitch muscle fibers will give you the power to perform the explosive moves.

In summary, you will build an aerobic base by doing sustained aerobic exercise such as power walking, jogging, or biking. Add fast aerobic exercise to increase power.

SIGNS OF OVERTRAINING

- Decreased performance
- Increased recovery needs
- Changes to resting heart rate
- Chronic fatigue
- Sleep disorders
- Eating disorders
- Menstrual disruptions
- Muscle soreness and damage
- Joint aches and pains
- Depression and apathy
- Increased illness
- Lowered self-esteem

Source: American College of Sports Medicine

THE CHALLENGE OF OVERCOMING INJURIES

When injury strikes, don't stop exercising. Modify your activity and keep going! Recently, while running, I tore the meniscus in my left knee, giving me considerable pain and leaving me limping around New York City. I made the usual visit to the orthopedic surgeon, had an MRI, and was told surgery was not indicated in my situation. But he advised me to have physical therapy and gradually my knee would heal. Instead of my usual running routine, I was forced to restrict myself to only a stationary bicycle. For any of you runners out there, you know it's just not the same! Gone was the endorphin-induced high! Sitting on a bike was just no fun and I really began to feel very sorry for myself. One day when I was on a bike at my gym, a man in an electric wheelchair entered, and proceeded to get up out of his chair with his back hunched over, slowly got on the treadmill, and started to walk at the very slowest speed. Gradually over the course of a few minutes, he was able to stand up straighter. He stayed on for a while longer, and when he finished, he got back into his chair. I said to him, "You're my new hero." He asked, "Why is that?" I explained that while many able-bodied people find excuses not to exercise, although he was in a wheelchair, he was motivated to get himself onto the treadmill. I explained to him that I am a physician who advocates exercise for her patients and as we chatted, he shared that he had multiple sclerosis (MS), which is a degenerative disease of the nervous system. He told me that he has a daily routine of treadmill for five minutes, and then he uses the ergometer for five minutes, and then he swims. I found this gentleman totally inspiring. When I entered the gym that morning, I was feeling sorry for myself because I couldn't run, and then I met a man with MS in a wheelchair who had the perseverance and strength to exercise.

My point is, you have to work with what you have. It is human nature to be upset by injury; stay positive and keep moving to overcome it.

LETTING OFF SOME STEAM

These clubs are where elite Manhattanites go to stay trim and fit. They offer steam rooms and a wonderful array of high-tech machines, well-designed programs, and trainers on site.

- Focus Integrated Fitness—Specializes in in-home personal training. The trainers all have multiple certifications and are required to attend ongoing training. This is the gold standard of in-home training. www.focusnyc.com
- David Barton Gym—www.davidbartongym.com
- Equinox Fitness Clubs—www.equinoxfitness.com
- The Sports Club/LA—www.thesportsclubla.com
- Clay—www.insideclay.com
- Madison Square Club—www.davidkirsh.com
- Uptown Pilates—Small luxurious Pilates studio with excellent instructors at 903 Madison Avenue on the Upper East Side of Manhattan. Mika Street is the owner. www.uptownpilates.com

---

THE FOUNTAIN OF YOUTH

The declines in physical performance that accompany aging include reduced muscle mass, increased percentage of body fat, poor balance, reduced respiratory capacity, and reduced cardiac output. All the changes that age imposes on the body can be postponed or improved with exercise. Likewise, they are worsened by inactivity. Inactivity causes blood pressure to rise and daily exercise will result in it becoming normal.

Muscle strength declines 7 percent per decade after age thirty unless we exercise. To maintain muscle strength, we need resistive exercise. That means weights, or we will become weak. If the muscles are not challenged they develop "disuse atrophy"; they shrink and lose their strength. High-quality protein in the diet helps to maintain strength.

Lisa is a sixty-two-year-old psychotherapist who came to see me because of her increasing waistline. Although naturally slim, over the last few years Lisa had noted that her clothes fit differently, particularly through the waistline. Lisa had always been a calorie-watcher, but did not particularly enjoy exercising, so she avoided it. In fact, Lisa's diet was quite limited, consisting of processed "low-calorie" foods and very little protein. A typical dinner for Lisa was a frozen low-fat, diet dinner. She reported that she felt "stiff" in the morning and both knees ached (a sure sign of arthritis). Of concern I noted that her total cholesterol was high, but the good HDL cholesterol was low. C-reactive protein, a measure of inflammation, was also high. Additionally, during the physical examination her blood pressure was noted to be borderline high at 135/80 and her waist size was thirty-seven inches, although her body weight was normal. She was a classic apple shape! Lisa was aging her body by an avoidance of exercise! She sat all day due to the sedentary nature of her job and was not doing her part to keep her body young. Her blood pressure and total cholesterol were too high. Her laboratory results indicated an alarming number of risk factors for cardiovascular disease: high LDL "bad" cholesterol, low HDL "good" cholesterol, and an elevated C-reactive protein (CRP). Additionally, Lisa's waist size was a risk factor—it is indicative of fat stored within the body cavity, deep behind the muscle. Often people have the mistaken idea that if they are not eating meat or butter or other known cholesterol-raising foods, they are safe. They are incorrect because a high-sugar or high-simple-carbohydrate diet causes the liver to produce cholesterol. The answer for Lisa was to change her diet and to make daily aerobic exercise a priority. Although she did not like the idea of exercise, she disliked the way she looked more and agreed to give exercise a try. Because of her painful knees, the stationary bicycle was her means of exercise and she faithfully pedaled for 30 minutes daily. Three times per week she followed a resistive exercise regime to strengthen her muscles. As time went by, she found that she actually looked forward to her exercise. She had less discomfort in her joints and began a walking program. Lisa began to feel better almost immediately. After six months, I repeated Lisa's laboratory work and found that her cholesterol and CRP had become normal. When I examined her, I found that Lisa's blood pressure was normal and that her waist size had gone down two inches (within the range of normal). Lisa had gone back to her health profile of fifteen years ago. She had become younger by exercising and by changing her diet to include youth-promoting foods.

Aerobic exercise is the foundation but not the whole story. For you to be in top form it is important to address both balance exercises and posture. Each of these elements contributes to fitness in a different way. It is not time consuming to add balance and posture training to an exercise routine. In fact, for balance training all you really need to do is practice standing on one leg with your eyes closed. While talking on the telephone or waiting for an elevator or a bus, just stand on one leg. To focus on posture while you are doing your errands or aerobic walk just say to yourself, "Shoulders back and down. Pull in your stomach." Bingo. You have it all.

BALANCE EXERCISE

As we age, it is essential that we practice balance activity daily. Older individuals who incorporate tai chi or yoga maintain their balance, have fewer falls, and fewer fractures. The main reason balance declines with age is lack of practice. Without stimulation the proprioceptive nerve fibers (which tell us where our limbs are in space) become less active, the muscles supplied by the fibers begin to atrophy, and we notice we are a "little unsteady." We don't use it so we lose it! The beauty of balance-promoting exercise is that you notice an improvement right away. Foods high in vitamin B complex help with balance by preserving our nerves.

POSTURE EXERCISE

My *newest* favorite exercise is Pilates; we even offer Pilates exercises in my Park Avenue practice. Joseph Pilates was a fitness enthusiast who felt that alignment was essential to moving correctly. He devised an interesting series of exercises on machines utilizing springs and ropes to strengthen the postural muscles. The muscles of posture include all the muscles between the chest and knees: abdominals, back, glutes, shoulders, quadriceps, and hamstrings. Weakness in any of these muscles is seen in the posture.

When I was a resident in rehabilitation medicine I witnessed just how intertwined the action of the postural muscles can be. In the stroke clinic I treated individuals who were recovering from the devastating damage that stroke can cause. Most strokes are caused by an obstruction in an artery in the brain. The damage that results is dependent on the area of the body that is controlled by the affected region of the brain. The most common stroke affects the left side of the brain, which controls the right side of the body. Once the patient has been stabilized, rehabilitation begins. The muscles of the face, arm, torso, and leg can be weakened. The shoulder muscles no longer dynamically hold the shoulder in its socket, it appears to hang in place. The back muscles on the affected side are weak; back pain is common. The hip muscles cannot support the pelvis and it drops on the affected side. The thigh muscles, responsible for flexing and extending the thigh during normal gait, have lost strength and walking becomes a challenge. While weakness in any one muscle interferes with movement, the importance of all the muscles in the chain working in coordination is dramatically seen in a stroke. Because it is the core muscles that support posture, gait and all movement activities are compromised.

Everyone should know the risks for a stroke, as they are for the most part conditions that can be prevented, or reversed, by diet and exercise. The risks are high blood pressure, smoking cigarettes, atherosclerosis, diabetes, and transient ischemic attack (when a brain artery is obstructed, but the obstruction spontaneously clears on its own).

Pilates addressed this interdependence of muscles affecting posture with his exercises which strengthen the core muscles.

QUICK PICK-ME-UPS

At the office increase your productivity with these anytime energizers:

- Sitting at your computer, remind yourself, "Suck your navel in to meet your backbone. Pull your shoulders back and down."
- Seated Cat and Cow: Sitting up straight, exhale as you tightly pull in your abdominal muscles and roll back onto your pelvis,

forming a big C curve. As you inhale reverse the curve. Slowly roll your pelvis and chest forward. Open up your chest and pull your shoulders back. Repeat several times.

- Stand with your back against a wall, pinching your shoulders back for ten seconds.
- Squeeze your butt as tightly as possible while talking on the phone.
- Before going into a meeting do neck rolls, followed by standing with your back against the wall; pull in your abdominal muscles and walk into the room with perfect posture and confidence.
- Don't let your fingers do the walking! Deliver all messages personally by walking to your colleagues; no more e-mails within the same office.
- Schedule walking meetings. This will keep your entire office energized! It will work best with groups of less than six employees. Many companies are now scheduling meetings in this manner. As a hospital resident, I looked forward to the morning rounds because of the updates of all patients under my care. The fact that we walked into each individual hospital room made the time quickly pass. Had we not made a point of individually visiting each patient, it would not have been nearly so informative or enjoyable!
- Try to leave your office building for at least a few minutes daily. A change of scene can make a big difference! Walk around the block with an energetic stride.

By the way, desk jobs are not good for you. Beside the inactivity that is imposed, think of the effect on posture. Your shoulders are slumped, your head is forward, and your chest sags. Your back is taking a major hit. During workouts at the gym, reverse the damage by concentrating on posture alignment with back-strengthening exercises. Avoid the exercise bike and get on the treadmill or, if your knees are bothering you, elliptical trainer. The elliptical trainer is a stationary exercise machine that simulates running without the stress of impact on the joints.

Somehow many people do not think of themselves as athletes. When I refer to my patients as athletes, they often chuckle and say, "Oh sure, that's a laugh." Yet they do consider individuals such as the Williams sisters or Tiger Woods to be athletes. In fact, if you asked them about these professional athletes they would probably say, "Of course. Are you crazy?" But I maintain that you and I are just as much athletes as those individuals who rake in the big bucks. What separates us, really? On a simple level we all move because of our muscles. You, me, Tiger Woods, Secretariat, all of us are able to move because of nerves and muscles. All share the same infrastructure, if you will. All muscles stay strong and healthy with exercise and become smaller and weaker without it.

We are able to move because our muscles contract. The contraction of muscles occurs because of amazing organs called mitochondria. Mitochondria can be thought of as an energy factory located within each muscle cell. Fueled by oxygen and either fat or glycogen, the mitochondria drive all motion.

Mitochondria explain why we breathe faster during exercise: They need a steady supply of oxygen.

FITNESS TEST

I. *Timed Sit-to-Stand Test.* This part will test the strength and endurance of the fast-twitch muscle fibers in the legs. To perform the test: Sit in the middle of a chair with a seat height of seventeen inches. The chair may be placed against the wall to prevent it from slipping. Keep your back straight, your feet flat on the floor, and your arms crossed on your chest. From this position, start the timer and rise to stand, return to sitting. Complete as many full stands as possible in thirty seconds. *Scoring:* Excellent is over 20, good is 20 to 15, poor is fewer than 15.[1]

2. *Balance Test.* Do you have good balance? Many people are surprised to see their balance isn't as good as they believed. Declines in balance are imperceptive until you have a fall. But the good news is that balance improves quickly with practice. Test your balance and if you need help, I've provided some exercises at the end of the chapter.

    Here is the test: On a smooth floor, stand barefoot on one leg with the other leg bent while keeping your eyes closed. Time yourself. Best out of three trials is used for score.

Scoring: An individual twenty years old should be able to stand for thirty seconds on one leg with eyes closed; a fifty-year-old should be able to stand for fifteen seconds with eyes closed.[2]

3. *Strength of Your Upper Body.* Do you know that fewer than 10 percent of women over the age of fifty can lift twenty pounds over their heads? In our daily lives we don't do very much overhead lifting. But what about when you board an airline and need to put your suitcase in the overhead compartment? Wouldn't it be gratifying to do that all on your own without having to ask for help? Let's start by testing your upper-body strength. Push-up test for men: Start in the standard position of hands pointing forward and under the shoulders, back straight, head in line with spine, legs straight, using the toes as the pivotal point. Push-up test for women: Use the modified knee push-up position of legs together, knees on the mat, back straight, hands shoulder width apart, head up, using the knees as the pivotal point. Lower the body to the down position until the chin almost touches the mat. For both men and women, the back must be straight at all times and you must push up to straight arm position. The maximum number of push-ups performed consecutively without rest is your score.

Scoring Females: Ages 20 to 29—excellent is 30 push-ups, good is 29 to 15, fair is 14 to 10. Ages 30 to 39—excellent is 27 push-ups, good is 26 to 13, fair is 12 to 8. Ages 40 to 49—excellent is 24 push-ups, good is 23 to 11, fair is 10 to 5. Ages 50 to 59—excellent is 21 push-ups, good is 20 to 11, and fair is 6 to 2. Ages 60 plus—excellent is 17 push-ups, good is 16 to 5, and fair is 4 to 2.

Scoring Males: Ages 20 to 29—excellent is 36 push-ups, good is 35 to 22, fair is 21 to 17. Ages 30 to 39—excellent is 30 push-ups, good is 29 to 17, fair is 16 to 12. Ages 40 to 49—excellent is 25, good is 24 to 13, fair is 12 to 10. Ages 50 to 59—excellent is 21 push-ups, good is 20 to 10, fair is 9 to 7. Ages 60 plus—excellent is 18, good is 17 to 8, fair is 7 to 5.[3]

4. *Abdominal Strength.* Do you have abs of steel? Few people do but you do require core strength to move efficiently without injury. Without good core strength, your back injury risk soars because the back muscles are recruited to do the work of the abdominals. Try this test: Lie on your

back with your hips and knees bent to ninety degrees and your feet off the ground. Cross your arms over your chest and keep your chin slightly tucked. Perform a slow, controlled curl to lift the shoulder blades off the mat (trunk makes a thirty-degree angle with the mat). Keep your lower back flat against the floor. Exhale while curling your upper body until just your shoulders are lifted. Don't come up to sitting! Return to start position. Do as many curls as possible in one minute.

Scoring: Excellent is 25, good is 24 to 12, and fair is 11 to 5.[4]

5. *Flexibility Test*. To move gracefully and reduce your risk for injury you need flexibility. And just how much flexibility you need is determined by what you do. By this I mean that a swimmer will require more flexibility of the shoulder than a runner. A gymnast will require more back and hip flexibility than a tennis player. The majority of us spend our time sitting, causing our hamstrings (the muscles in the back of the leg) and the connective tissue to become shorter as we age. We have trouble touching our toes. Take this test to assess your lower-back and hip-joint flexibility: Secure a yardstick to the floor by placing a twelve-inch length of tape across it at the ruler's fifteen-inch mark. Sit on the floor with the yardstick between your legs. With your legs extended, place one heel on each end of the taped line, about ten to twelve inches apart. Slowly reach forward with both hands as far as possible, while exhaling and dropping your head between your arms while reaching. Hold the position for two seconds. Be sure that your hands are kept parallel and do not lead with one hand. Look at the number on the yardstick that your hands reach.

Scoring: Excellent is 20 or above, good is 19 to 15, fair is 14 to 10.[5]

Now you have taken the test and gotten "excellent" in every category. Congratulations! You have reached a fabulous level of fitness and you have my admiration. But for the rest of us, all the test has done is identify areas that we can improve.

Following is a workout that I designed with my trainer, Joe Masiello, of Focus Integrated Fitness, New York City. Joe says that the best all-around exercise is the push-up. He says that it engages the upper and lower body. He puts the push-up into all our sessions.

The idea is to get you going and to exercise all muscle groups. Put on some music or tune in to energizing music on your iPod and unleash your inner athlete:

1. Warm up for fifteen to twenty minutes with a fast walk or dance. Always warm up before you work out. You do not need to stretch before working out and may injure yourself if you stretch before your muscles are warmed up. As you walk be aware of your posture and hold your shoulders back and down. After you have finished your warm-up give yourself a balance challenge: Stand on one leg, focus on your posture, and then close your eyes. Maintain the position for as long as you can, then challenge yourself on the other leg.

2. Legs. Work out your legs first because they are the largest muscle groups; your warm-up has gotten them primed for exercise. Using a chair, with your arms crossed over your chest, squat until your bottom touches the seat, then stand. Repeat for two sets of ten repetitions.

3. Arms. Start with bicep curls using a five-pound with weight in each hand, keep your elbows tucked into your sides and positioned under your shoulders, and keep your shoulders back and down. If five pounds is too heavy for you, start with three-pound weights—don't worry, you will get stronger. Do two sets of ten repetitions. After a few days, when you are comfortable with the exercise, try it standing on a Bosu or a balance board to build your balance. By incorporating balance here you are working efficiently. Next, using five-pound weights, with your elbows bent ninety degrees and at your sides, raise the weights overhead and extend your arms. Repeat for two sets of ten repetitions. Do not practice balance with this exercise and stop this exercise if you experience shoulder pain.

4. Chest. By doing this exercise on a stability ball you will increase your core strength and balance. Stability balls are large inflatable plastic balls that you can sit on. Sitting on a stability ball requires you to activate your abdominal muscles to maintain your balance. I highly recommend them. (If you do not have a stability ball, you can perform the exercise lying on the floor with your knees bent.)

Lying on your back across an inflated stability ball, position yourself so that your upper back and chest are supported by the ball and your knees are bent ninety degrees. Keep your abdominals tightened. Using five-pound weights in each hand, extend them directly over your chest until your arms are straight. Do two sets of ten repetitions.

5. Abdominals. Lying on your back with your hips and knees bent ninety degrees, cross your arms over your chest, slightly tuck your chin, and use your abdominals to raise your shoulders off the mat. Repeat twenty times. The goal here is to make your abdominal muscles stronger so they will protect your back. When you can comfortably do twenty repetitions, increase until you can do fifty.

6. Back extensions. Any woman with reduced bone density is advised to do this exercise. Lying on your stomach on the mat, lift a straight leg and the opposite arm, repeat with the other leg and arm. Count this as one repetition (using right and left once each). Do two sets of ten repetitions.

7. End with a challenge to your balance by standing on one leg with your eyes closed, then repeat on the other leg.

8. Complete your workout with a good stretch. Lie on your back, with your arms out to the sides. Bring your knees in to your chest and let them fall to the right side of the body. Keep your torso straight and breathe deeply. Repeat on left. This stretches back and hip muscles. Next, lying with your feet on the floor and your knees bent, extend your right leg overhead. Hold the stretch by pulling in a towel wrapped around your calf. Repeat on the left. This stretches your hamstring muscles.

This workout is a suggestion to get you started. It works all major muscle groups and will serve to introduce you to the wonderful world of fitness. After you have mastered the workout, in a couple of weeks, you must join a gym. Joining a gym gives you a whole new opportunity for getting stronger and energetic. The energy of the gym will boost your spirits on the days when you just don't want to exercise.

WORKOUT ENERGY PLEASER

OMEGA-3 FRUITY SMOOTHIE
Use a miniblender, and swirl together my Everyday Nutrition vanilla shake with one-half cup of blueberries or strawberries, or an Everyday Nutrition chocolate shake with ½ cup cherries for a delicious quick smoothie to perk you out of an afternoon slump so you can get to the gym!

EXERCISING IN THE BIG APPLE

These are some of my favorite New York sites for a great workout:

- *Biking Your Way on New York's Bridges*—We have the Brooklyn, the Queensborough, and the Triborough, for starters.
- *Central Park*—Central Park is my ultimate fitness haunt, and where I often begin my day. For as many years as I have lived in New York, I always seem to discover something new and exciting in the park. It offers a virtual smorgasbord of exercise attractions including skating in Wollman Memorial Skating Rink and practicing your serve at the Central Park Tennis Center. I especially enjoy going through the park in the morning before the city awakes. Early in the morning the park is a green paradise, surrounded by granite spires of towering office and apartment buildings. You are in the city and yet out of the city at the same time. Shakespeare Garden, the reservoir, the Conservatory Garden, and the Harlem Meer are just a few of the beautiful spots. www.centralpark.com
- *Battery Park*—What a great place to start or end your run! The scenery is amazing.
- *Carl Schurz Park*—The East River views from this charming park delight young and old alike. Situated right next door to Gracie Mansion, where New York's mayors have lived, the park is a perfect spot for running next to the East River, rollerblading among the trees, playing

hoops, taking your kids to the monkey bars, or pushing your baby in a swing. There are even two dog runs: one fenced patch for large breeds, and a concrete playground just for the toy and puppy set under twenty pounds. The East River has a jogging path that leads all the way to the tip of Manhattan.

- *Riverside Park*—Known as a hangout for intellectuals, this park lies on the Upper West Side of Manhattan.
- *Chelsea Piers*—A unique urban playground complex for adults and children, this twenty-eight-acre megastructure is located on the Hudson River. There is something for everyone here: the best bowling lanes in Manhattan, gymnastics, and dance classes of all kinds, Olympic-sized pools, a golf club, soccer programs, a comprehensive sports center, rock climbing, the Sky Rink for skaters, and the Bluestreak Sports Training Center. www.chelseapiers.com

CHAPTER NINE

THE SLEEP FACTOR

Whate'er thy joys, they vanish with the
day: Whate'er thy griefs, in sleep they
fade away, To sleep! To sleep! Sleep,
mournful heart, and let the past be past.

—ALFRED LORD TENNYSON,
"FORESTER'S SONG"

Are you a night owl? Or are you the early bird in your family who wakes everyone else up?

HEALTHY BENEFITS OF SLEEP

Every evening between 9:30 and 10 P.M. I begin preparing for bed. I take a relaxing bath, arrange my papers for the next day, do a few balance and stretching exercises, and then I climb into bed. Although there is a television in our bedroom, my husband and I listen to it only while getting ready for work in the morning. We prefer to keep our bedroom quiet and peaceful at night. We make it a point to avoid discussions that might turn into arguments after dinner. I am a "good sleeper" and do not require a sleeping pill. I wake up at 5:30 A.M. without an alarm clock, ready to begin a new day.

I give you my own formula for successful sleep, as I do with my patients, because they work for most people. But not all people. Executives with extensive travel schedules, students with evening classes, new parents, and others may need to modify some of the principles. But the key principles hold. For you to work at your peak and to feel your best, you must rest your body well.

The importance of getting enough sleep on a nightly basis (instead of just occasionally) cannot be overstated. Sleep is essential for your body to renew itself. Sleep deprivation is cumulative; so if you are missing sleep night after night, the effects will eventually catch up with you.

While the precise amount of sleep needed for optimal functioning varies from person to person, the average amount is seven to eight hours per night. Your body needs to recharge, and this is only possible if you get enough rest on a regular basis. Food cannot compensate for a lack of sleep. In fact, the less you sleep, the more difficult it is for your body to digest food. So be sure to get the right combination with regular meals *and* regular sleeping patterns.

HOW MUCH SLEEP DO YOU NEED?

When I talk with my patients about sleep, I ask these questions:

1. **Do you have a regular bedtime?** By going to bed at the same time every night, you teach your body that it is time to sleep. Your body comes to expect that it will sleep at that time. It becomes more efficient at falling asleep.
2. **Do you avoid caffeine and alcohol in the evening?** Caffeine has a half-life of approximately nine hours. Half-life is how we determine how long a drug stays in the body. After nine hours, half of the caffeine you consumed has been metabolized. For some people, including me, coffee after 3 P.M. in the afternoon is not a good idea. Alcohol makes us sleepy but after several hours it can cause awakening.
3. **Do you have a method of preparing yourself for sleep?** A warm bath or listening to a relaxing piece of music are ways to tell the body that sleep will soon occur. A prominent designer in New York City has a massage nightly that is so relaxing to her, the masseuse tiptoes out after her client has fallen into a deep sleep.

4. **Is your bedroom quiet, dark, and cool?** Noise and light are stimuli to awaken.

5. **Is your mattress comfortable?** Who could possibly enjoy sleep on a substandard mattress? Do not compromise on your mattress. Take the time to test it in the store. Buy the best.

The physical steps that you take in preparing for sleep can make the difference between tossing and turning and getting the restful sleep that is needed.

Joan was the chief financial officer of a clothing manufacturer, and she was recruited to head up another clothing firm that was much farther away from her home. When I met her, she had a terrible commute of two hours from Connecticut to Manhattan each way. She left her house every morning at 6 A.M. and a driver picked her up to take her to work every day. Her biggest problem was that she worked late into the night on her computer, often not going to bed until 1 A.M. She was sleeping barely four hours nightly! Joan was also suffering from terrible migraines. Botox injections helped somewhat, and her neurologist had even prescribed narcotics to help ease the debilitating pain. After I evaluated her lifestyle more closely, I learned that Joan fell asleep in the car going to work every day, in an attempt to make up the sleep she wasn't getting during the night. Joan's laboratory results revealed high levels of insulin, cortisol, and cholesterol. Her physical exam showed her blood pressure to be borderline high at 135/80mm/Hg with a pulse of eighty bpm. Joan's lack of sleep meant she was perpetually in a state of stress, as indicated by her high insulin and cortisol levels.

I emphasized to Joan the importance of sleep and gave her a schedule for increasing her sleep at night. I asked her to be in bed by 12:30 A.M. for the next three nights while avoiding sleeping on the way to work. She was to move her bedtime back by thirty minutes every evening until she was in bed by 10 P.M. Additionally, she was instructed to exercise

every morning on her treadmill for thirty minutes. Besides depriving herself of sleep, Joan was also depriving herself of daily exercise! Sleep and
exercise are two proven remedies for stress. So she changed her patterns,
and instead of napping in the backseat, she worked on her BlackBerry,
and went to bed right after 10 P.M. Joan immediately did well with the
plan and saw a reduction in the number of migraines. She has had a few
slipups but because she is now conscious of the effect sleep has on her
body, she gets back on track. This worked brilliantly for about a year,
until Joan decided that she had enough of the commute and made a
change in her life. She ultimately became a consultant, which allowed her
much more freedom and gave her more time to spend with her husband,
eliminating the commute and the late-night workload. The last time I
saw Joan, she was relaxed, the migraines were gone, and she was toned
and trim because she had taken up swimming, which she loved.

ENERGY PEARL

If you suspect that you are sleep deprived, move your bedtime up by
thirty minutes but continue to get up at the same time. Do not try to
fix your sleep debt by sleeping later. Every three days go to bed another thirty minutes earlier until you are getting the right amount of
sleep for your body.

GETTING A GOOD NIGHT'S SLEEP

Women are more likely than men to have sleep disturbance due to anxiety or depression, whereas
men are twice as likely to have sleep apnea than women.

Women report more sleeping disorders than men. I suspect this is because of
our hormonal fluctuations involving estrogen. It is well known that women experience difficulty with sleep around their periods, during pregnancy, and when
they are going through menopause. Thyroid disturbances can cause alterations in

sleep; hypothyroidism causes excessive sleep and hyperthyroidism causes insomnia. Chronic fatigue disorder and mood disorders affect sleep phases as well. Depression, especially winter depression, often causes sleep disruptions. Changes in your daily schedule and environment due to travel or traffic noises and other disturbances wreak havoc on your sleep patterns. Medical conditions that cause pain or aches like toothaches, or sleep apnea also contribute to the problem.

FIVE TIPS FOR BEATING INSOMNIA

1. Avoid stimulants like caffeine and nicotine, painkillers, coffee, tea, prescription drugs.
2. For the few hours before bedtime, keep the lights low in the living room and in the bedroom.
3. Put a lavender-scented sachet under your pillow; it is a natural sleep inducer.
4. Late-night eating can disturb your sleep since the body stays awake as food is digested. Hunger pangs may also keep you awake if you go to bed on an empty stomach.
5. Stress and anxiety keep you from falling asleep when your mind is too active thinking about work, money, or health problems. Worrying about getting to sleep can make it hard to fall asleep!

TYPES OF SLEEP

Deep sleep is not reached when you have too many interruptions in your sleep time. An occasional catnap may be beneficial if you need it, but sleeping for a few hours during the day may just make you feel more tired.

THE SLEEP STEALERS

RESTLESS LEGS SYNDROME

RLS is a common sleep disorder estimated to affect 9 percent of Americans. RLS is characterized by a "creepy crawly" feeling in the legs that is relieved by moving. It appears in the evening and worsens after bedtime. RLS can even awaken an individual from sleep! Pain is not a usual component. Sleep is disrupted and daytime lethargy results. The prevalence in women is twice that of men, so the true prevalence in women is estimated to be as high as 16 percent.[1] It is likely that estrogen increases the tendency for RLS as the incidence during pregnancy is two to three times that of nonpregnant women.

RLS should send you right to your doctor's office because it may be a symptom of illness. Your doctor will do blood tests to rule out iron deficiency anemia, diabetes, and kidney disease. These conditions will worsen if not treated and RLS may improve as underlying conditions are treated.

If your sleep is disturbed by RLS, first attempt to control the condition by changing your behavior:

- Avoid alcohol.
- Do not smoke.
- Drink caffeine only in the morning.
- Exercise daily in moderate amounts.
- Take a hot bath before bed.
- Take at least 50mg magnesium every evening.

Mild and moderate cases of RLS usually are improved by following these suggestions, and more severe cases may be treated with medications. There are two prescription medications that may help: Mirapex and Requip. Alternatively, antiseizure medications and opiates may help.

LEG CRAMPS

Cramps in the legs that occur at night should not be confused with RLS. The cramps occur in the calves and are painful. The muscle will become tense for anywhere from fifteen seconds to ten minutes. Leg cramps usually represent an electrolyte imbalance caused by dehydration. Make sure that you are drinking enough water. If dehydration isn't the problem, you might try magnesium supplements to relieve the pain.

CHRONIC FATIGUE SYNDROME

Chronic fatigue syndrome (CFS) affects more than one million people in the United States. According to the Centers for Disease Control and Prevention (CDC), less than 20 percent of CFS patients have been diagnosed. There are millions of people with similar fatigue-inducing illnesses who do not fully meet the strict definition of CFS.

CFS is a debilitating and complex disorder characterized by profound fatigue that is not improved by bed rest and may be worsened by physical or mental activity. People with CFS often function at a lower level of activity than they were capable of before the onset of illness. Patients also report various nonspecific symptoms, including weakness, muscle pain, impaired memory and/or mental concentration, insomnia, and postexertional fatigue lasting more than twenty-four hours. In some cases, CFS can persist for years. The cause or causes of CFS have not been identified and no specific diagnostic tests are available. Moreover, since many illnesses have incapacitating fatigue as a symptom, it is often hard to exclude other conditions when making a diagnosis of CFS.

The clinical measure of CFS involves two criteria:

1. A patient must have severe chronic fatigue of six months or longer duration with other known medical conditions excluded by clinical diagnosis.
2. Concurrently the patient must have four or more of the following symptoms: substantial impairment in short-term memory or concentration; sore throat; tender lymph nodes; muscle pain; multijoint pain without swelling or redness; headaches of a new type, pattern, or severity; unrefreshing sleep; and postexertional malaise lasting more than twenty-four hours.

The symptoms must have persisted or recurred during six or more consecutive months of illness and must not have predated the fatigue.

HOW TO TELL IF YOU MAY HAVE CFS

There are no physical signs that identify CFS. People who suffer the symptoms of CFS must be carefully evaluated by a physician because many treatable medical and psychiatric conditions are hard to distinguish from CFS.

GETTING TREATMENT

Since there is no known cure for CFS, treatment is aimed at symptom relief and improved function. No single therapy exists that helps all CFS patients. Lifestyle changes, including preventing overexertion, reducing stress, improving diet and nutrition, and stretching are frequently recommended in addition to drug therapies used to treat sleep disorders, pain, and other specific symptoms.

FAST FACTS ABOUT CFS

- CFS affects women at four times the rate of men.
- CFS is most common in people in their forties and fifties.
- Although CFS is much less common in children than in adults, teens can develop it.

OTHER SLEEP DISRUPTERS

- Neurological conditions—especially those affecting movement—usually impact on sleep patterns—Parkinson's disease, multiple sclerosis.
- Headache.
- Gastrointestinal disturbances.
- Pregnancy.

Leslie is a thirty-five-year-old account executive who has risen to the top in a highly competitive field of advertising in a major New York advertising firm. Leslie is slim and energetic due to her five-year habit of 5:30 A.M. workouts at the gym. She is in her office by 7 A.M., organizing her day with efficient lists. Her e-mails are answered and at the 9 A.M. meeting she updates her sales team on the priorities of the day. Her workday often extends into the evening as she entertains clients in New York City chic spots. But her motto is "Early to bed, early to rise," and she hits the sack at 9:30 or 10 P.M. Her personal life is rich with many friends, a close family relationship, and a loving relationship with her new husband. Intelligent and inquisitive, Leslie can converse on politics, contemporary art, history, and Hollywood gossip with clarity and wit. She is boundless in her love of life. In short, she appears to be someone who has it all. Leslie has organized her sleep to promote energy.

MEDICATIONS THAT AFFECT SLEEP

- Steroidal medications
- Birth control
- Asthma medication
- Antidepressants
- Nicotine replacement patches
- Thyroid medications
- Stimulants taken to treat ADD

THE DANGERS OF SLEEPING PILLS

Sedatives, also called tranquilizers, work by depressing the central nervous system to produce a calming or relaxing effect. Sedatives can be abused to produce an overly calming effect, as in alcohol abuse. At high doses, some of these drugs can cause unconsciousness and even death. All sedatives can cause physiological and psychological dependence when taken regularly over a period of time. When users become psychologically dependent, they feel as if they need the drug to function even though there is no biological dependence. Ambien (Sanofi-Aventis), Sonata (King Pharmaceuticals), and Lunesta (Sepracor) are the top-selling sleeping pills in the United States.

HERBAL SEDATIVES

Looking for something to help you sleep that won't leave you groggy and hungover? There are herbal approaches to helping you sleep. I hesitate to recommend them unilaterally because the science just isn't there. We need controlled trials to demonstrate proof. But I will tell you anecdotally that I have met people who swear by them. Try these healthy herbal alternatives to get a good night's rest.

- Valerian is an herbal that may help when taken at bedtime.
- A glass of skim milk—old-fashioned as it sounds, it's comforting and many say induces sleep.
- Melatonin capsules taken just before retiring are said, it's help with jet lag and insomnia.

Are You in Sleep Debt?

The need for sleep varies with each individual. The average is seven to eight hours a night. If you do not satisfy your requirement, a sleep debt accumulates. As an example, say your requirement is seven hours but on Monday night you sleep only six hours, this means you have a sleep debt of one hour. If this continues through the week, by Friday night you will have accumulated a five-hour sleep debt. With a sleep debt you feel tired and uninspired. You just don't have the same intensity as you did on Monday morning. I hear this very frequently from my patients.

Balance your sleep just as you balance your checkbook and stay out of debt!

MEASURING YOUR DEBT

If you suspect you are not sleeping adequately, evaluate your sleep debt with the following test.

EPWORTH SLEEPINESS SCALE

How likely are you to doze off or fall asleep in the following situations? Score
    yourself according to the following scale:

0=would never doze

1=slight chance of dozing

2=moderate chance of dozing

3=high chance of dozing

Sitting and reading. _____

Watching TV. _____

Sitting quietly in a public place, such as on a bus or in a
    meeting. _____

As a passenger in a car for an hour without a break. _____

Lying down for a rest in the afternoon when circumstances
    allow. _____

Sitting and talking to someone. _____

Sitting quietly after lunch (no alcohol consumed). _____

In a car, while stopped for a few minutes in traffic. _____

TOTAL SCORE_____

Evaluate your total score.

0 to 5 Slight or no sleep debt

6 to 10 Moderate sleep debt

11 to 20 Heavy sleep debt

21 to 25 Extreme sleep debt

Any score over 6 should be promptly addressed. You need sleep and cannot
vigorously function while you are in sleep debt. And if you are driving an auto-
mobile you are endangering your own safety and that of others.

It is crucial that we sleep adequately, whatever our individual need. My own
need is just about seven hours. I admire people who are able to function optimally on three or four hours. I wish I could. But since I can't, I try to get the
sleep my body requires. It isn't always easy. Sometimes I feel like a wet blanket,
especially when others are having a great time. The good thing about New

York is that everyone has a unique schedule and leaving early is generally accepted.

THE ART OF THE NAP

*Nature had not intended mankind to work
from eight in the morning until midnight
without the refreshment of blessed
oblivion which, even if it lasts twenty
minutes, is sufficient to renew all the
vital forces.*

—SIR WINSTON CHURCHILL

If you are unable to get a good night's rest, a short nap can be a good idea. Call it a "Disco Nap" as one of my club-going friends does, or a "Power Nap." Just don't sleep longer than twenty minutes or your sleep pattern will suffer. To sleep longer than twenty minutes risks sleep inertia. Sleep inertia is when you awaken from your nap feeling exhausted rather than refreshed. It occurs because you allowed your nap to extend into deep sleep. Because sleep stages one and two are light stages of sleep and together last only twenty minutes, a nap of this duration is optimal. During stage one we sink into sleep, respiration slows, pulse and blood pressure fall, and our muscles relax. In stage two we relax more deeply, core temperature falls and the body begins to prepare itself for entry into deep sleep. Beyond twenty minutes, you enter stages three and four with deep, dreamless sleep where the muscles are paralyzed and brain waves slow, followed by REM (rapid eye movement).

You can either sleep for twenty minutes or allow extra time to complete slow wave sleep, with a ninety-minute sleep. So your choice is to nap for twenty minutes or ninety minutes—but nothing in between—and avoid sleep inertia. A nap can be refreshing during the times when you are under stress and sleep-deprived. It is not even necessary to lie down. I know several executives who just ask their secretaries to hold their telephone calls for thirty minutes when they lower the office lights and recline back in their desk chairs or rest their heads on their desks. A nap recharges their batteries and increases their energy.

ENERGY NAPPING

---

1. Recognize that the nap will increase your productivity and alertness. See the nap as an investment of time that will give you more energy. Realize that you are not being lazy!

2. Alert those around you that you are not to be disturbed. Empty your bladder. Turn the phones off and draw the shades. Darkness stimulates the production of melatonin, the sleep chemical.

3. Cover yourself in a light blanket. Body temperature falls during sleep and you want to optimally relax.

4. Once you are in position, set your alarm for twenty minutes.

Fatigue and Seasonal Affective Disorder (SAD)

SAD may account for the overwhelming desire we have to go into hibernation as the winter draws near. Accompanied by a marked decrease in energy, Seasonal Affective Disorder creeps up on people as the weather becomes cooler and the sun sets earlier in the day. Symptoms may include low mood, poor energy, lack of desire to be active, loss of sex drive, sadness, crying, inability to focus, and binge eating.

The best ways to conquer SAD is to let in the light. If you suffer from SAD, lighten your mood by getting some sun. Take a weekend trip to a warm, sunny place to perk you up. A change of scenery, even for a few days, can restore your mood to its former state of cheeriness. Energizing workouts or meditation may also improve your mood. Phototherapy uses artificial light to simulate the sun's positive psychological effects. The light should be 10,000 lux minimum. SSRI antidepressants are often prescribed to help you through the difficult months, but only as a last resort.

The M Word

Are your hormones keeping you up?

Menopause is a natural part of a woman's life. Technically, it marks the end of periods or menstrual cycle. The average age is about fifty-two; however, a woman's menopause can occur from ages thirty-five to sixty-five. Perimenopause is usually the two to five years before full menopause begins, but women may experience symptoms for a decade before stopping their periods. When symptoms arise at a young age it is commonly called early menopause. Symptoms can range from mild hot spells at night to constant dripping sweats all day and night. The symptoms are caused by hormonal imbalances and changes and are also related to diet and lifestyle. For most women, the menopause phase lasts from two to five years, although in some cases, it may seem like it's never going to end.

Some of my patients approach their fifties while working nonstop, caring for their children, husbands, and parents, and having almost no time left to take care of themselves. In short, they are burned out even before they hit menopause. When their diminishing estrogen meets hormonal turbulence, they find it hard to cope with all these changes thrown at them at once. The end result is that they have no reserve left to deal with this physically and emotionally difficult period in their lives when the body craves more rest.

Hormonal Highs and Lows—Symptoms of Menopause:

- Fatigue
- Cravings for sweets, carbs
- Weight gain
- Hot flashes
- Night sweats
- Depression
- Insomnia
- Anxiety
- Joint pain
- Irritable bowel
- Headaches
- Vaginal dryness
- Skin sagging
- Hair loss

Menopause can bring on migraines, restlessness, and sleep disturbances in the form of night sweats and hot flashes. It can also cause women to feel angry and depressed, feelings they sometimes take out on the people closest to them.

WORK SCHEDULES TAKE A TOLL

If your work schedule is constantly changing, you may feel tired most of the time. The level of the brain chemical serotonin drops in those who work days and nights on a fluctuating schedule, according to a study conducted by the Universidad de Buenos Aires in Argentina. The study found increased serotonin in those who worked during daylight hours as compared to those who worked both days and nights on a shifting basis. This chemical deficiency not only contributes to disrupted sleep cycles, but may also take a toll on your energy level, your mood, and your performance on the job.

Source: American Academy of Sleep Medicine, August 1, 2007

CHAPTER TEN

LIVE LONGER, LOOK YOUNGER

What you consume on a daily basis is as important to your health as what you do not consume. The adage "You are what you eat" certainly rings true for a generation that is bombarded with fast food, frozen entrées, and packaged food used for weight loss. Most Americans are too busy to prepare home-cooked meals and opt for convenience over nutrition. Not only does this affect your internal health, it affects the largest organ in your body—the skin. What you consume reveals itself in the quality and integrity of your skin. During the summer months, your skin is noticeable more than ever, as this is the time of year when you tend to wear less clothing. Undoubtedly exercise, specifically strength training, has a great impact on how you look in your swimsuit. However, the skin on your face and even your body, when not hiding behind a tan (real or sprayed on), divulges to the world how old you really are.

What steps can you institute right now to improve the quality of your skin? To begin with, change your diet. Research demonstrates that the consumption of sugary carbohydrate wreaks havoc on your skin. The reduction of carbohydrate in your daily menu will eliminate a source of damage and inflammation. Consumption of excess sugars results in the sugar attaching to the protein in your cells, creating a process called glycation. This process alters the structure of proteins all over your body. A high level of glucose in the blood causes inflammation as well. When circulating glucose attaches to collagen, it causes it to stiffen and results in sagging skin. Your body becomes damaged at the cellular level and the signs of aging such as wrinkled dry skin, brittle nails, and loss of skin tone contribute to making you appear older than you are. You can take all the supplements you want for weight loss and increased metabolism and have liposuction, but your skin does not lie. A lean body with sagging, wrinkled skin is not a youthful body. The key is to prevent aging of the skin by a diet of lean protein, essential fatty acids, and low glycemic carbohydrate.

My list of top foods for internal and external health is based on this concept. These foods, when consumed—along with cardiovascular conditioning and strength training—will transform your physique into a lean, toned, body that you will be proud to display during the summer and the remainder of the year.

TOP FOODS FOR INTERNAL AND EXTERNAL BEAUTY

1) *All green, leafy vegetables.* The darker the green, the better. They contain the power molecules, antioxidants, and essential omega and fatty acids.

2) *Organic eggs.* Eggs are a great source of complete protein and Mother Nature's perfect food. Eggs are rich in vitamin E, vitamin A, and choline, a nutrient important for the brain and nervous system. Dietary cholesterol like the kind you find in eggs has no impact on serum cholesterol. Dr. Walter Willett, chairman of the department of nutrition at the Harvard School of Public Health and a professor at Harvard Medical School, has said, "No research has ever shown that people who eat more eggs have more heart attacks than people who eat few eggs."

3) *Broccoli and other brassicas* (cauliflower, cabbage, Brussels sprouts). These vegetables are high in sulforaphane and indole-3 carbinol, which has been linked to prevention of cancers of the breast, uterus, prostate, and cervix. Also, all are low in glycemic value.

4) *Berries* (strawberries, raspberries, blueberries). All berries (preferably organic)

provide antioxidant protection and also contain ellagic acid, which is protective against cancer. All berries are low in glycemic value.

5) *Wild Alaskan salmon.* A great source of high-quality protein and one of the best sources of omega-3 fatty acids, beneficial for your heart, brain, anti-inflammatory response, circulation, memory, thought, and blood-sugar control.

6) *Nuts* (preferably raw and unroasted). Good sources of protein and essential fatty acids, fiber, and magnesium. Consumption of nuts has demonstrated a reduction in cholesterol, and may reduce the risk of heart disease. (Almonds are at the top of my list for their relationship to lowering heart disease and preventing cancer, and walnuts contain the highest amount of omega fats of any other nuts and they aid in brain functioning.)

7) *Extra virgin olive oil.* Acts as a natural anti-inflammatory. Consumption of olive oil is associated with a reduced risk of heart disease, stroke, heart and cardiovascular disease, breast cancer, lung cancer, and some forms of dementia.

8) *Kale.* A superstar with its high level of antioxidants and powerful cancer-fighting indoles and plant compounds, which have demonstrated their protective effect against breast, cervical, and colon cancer.

9) *Fish oil.* Good for the heart, brain, and skin. Inflammation generally manifests itself as rosacea, acne, psoriasis, or any kind of redness. It's also excellent for cardiovascular and brain function, inflammation and redness in the eyes, and supports healthy joints.

Blanche, a well-respected author, came to see me. She had been married later in life and had a child at age forty. In order to get pregnant, she had taken fertility drugs, which had caused weight gain. Her sedentary lifestyle as a writer did not help, either. I gave her a diet and exercise plan and she tried to stick to it, but she just couldn't lose weight. She was taking care of her adorable child and writing all the time, but neglected herself. With a hectic schedule like hers, she needed all the energy she could get. Traveling all the time from the East Coast to the West Coast, with frequent trips to Europe in between, was draining her and left her short-tempered with her daughter. Blanche got so busy that she could not come in to see me for six months. When she finally returned to my office, I didn't know what to expect. However, I was pleasantly surprised that she had kept her weight stable, and had not missed one day of going out for her daily run in the morning. She managed to do it all, and as her energy increased, she found that she could do more without feeling lethargic. Not only did she keep her weight down, but her husband lost twenty pounds, too.

YOUNG IN MIND AND SPIRIT, TOO

Age is mind over matter. If you don't mind, it doesn't matter.

—SATCHEL PAIGE

To maintain high energy, your mind needs to be sharp. You need to think clearly and with focus. Undoubtedly, what everyone fears is the loss of mental acuity that is thought to be associated with aging. Age-related dementia causes loss of memory and slowing of cognition. But what causes the change that occurs within the brain? Does the brain simply wear out with time? Why are some individuals so bright and engaged throughout their lives while other seniors seem to fade?

BRAIN DECLINE

An active area of research today is how brain tissue changes with age. As in all bodily processes, there are genes that control the changes in the brain. Identification of age-related brain changes and the genes responsible for them have been targeted as key research targets.

Genes that govern *plasticity*, or how new learning paths are built, are extremely active in childhood. When we are young, it is easier for us to learn a language. Perhaps the reason the paths are so active in childhood is this is when we need to learn so much. We come into the world as a blank canvas. Our immature brains are flooded with information from our senses. To organize the information, genes instruct sensory information to go to a specific brain region.

Sensory information from the eye is transmitted to the visual cortex, where it is stored. Soon, we are able to associate a visual image, such as the sight of our mother's face, with feeding. The reason we make these associations is because the genes governing the directing of sensory information cause the paths to be established. This represents plasticity; the genes that govern this enable us to learn new things throughout life.

AGE FORTY IS THE FORK IN THE ROAD

Dr. Bruce Yankner at Harvard found that in the early adult years (twenty-one to forty) brains show similar patterns of wear and tear and low levels of damage. After age seventy and older, brains exhibit recognizable damage. Looking at the genes of memory and learning, it would be impossible to mistake an old brain for a young one. There is "sameness" to both young and old brains. Young brains look young; old brains look old. But the really interesting finding is that between ages forty and seventy brains exhibit wide variations in aging. Middle age would seem to be the turning point. Some brains are virtually identical to the young brain, while others begin to show the beginnings of deleterious change. Changes seem to occur genetically before they are evident. Early changes in the gene plasticity and the gene's ability to repair itself precedes mental decline. It appears that oxidative stress damages the genes that enable us to learn and establish new paths in our brains. "Thus, our findings raise the exciting possibility that lifestyle changes in young adults could delay cognitive declines and protect against the onset of brain diseases in later years," Dr. Yankner concluded.

The majority of brain decline occurs in the genes governing learning and memory, according to Dr. Yankner. Alterations in these important genes can begin to appear by age forty. The young adult and older-aged brains have similarities in gene condition with the younger age demonstrating little damage. However, the tissue of the middle-age brain exhibits a wide variety of changes, with some brains appearing remarkably young and others aging more rapidly.

PREVENTION

Clearly, the trick is to prevent oxidative damage to the learning and memory genes before age forty when they seem to start their downhill descent. The principles of protecting against oxidative stress in the brain should be initiated early in life, in childhood. It is a wonder that we are so casual when it comes to feeding children, as though their young bodies can recuperate from any assault thrown at them. High-sugar, artificially sweetened, and high-fat foods cause oxidative stress in the body. Children have repair genes that help them to stay ahead of the damage somewhat. But why subject them to the harm in the first place?

The Mediterranean diet has been found to be associated with a low risk of cognitive decline and Alzheimer's disease. A recent four-year study by Columbia University followed 2,258 elderly individuals living in Manhattan. They tracked various components of Mediterranean eating:

- High intake of vegetables, fruit, fish, and legumes.
- Low amount of saturated fat, or animal fat, and higher amounts of unsaturated fat, such as that found in olive oil.
- Moderate alcohol consumption, preferably in the form of red wine.

What they found was that the more closely an individual followed the Mediterranean diet, the lower his or her risk for Alzheimer's disease. The one third of the individuals who followed the diet most closely had a 39 to 40 percent lower risk of Alzheimer's than the group that followed the more American-style diet. The interesting fact here is that they were elderly individuals living in the midst of Manhattan, where stress is high and they were surrounded by poor food choices—but healthful eating patterns protected them. They had learned these eating habits early in life, allowing the plasticity genes of memory and learning to remain active.

The Mediterranean diet gives high amounts of B vitamins and polyphenols, both of which protect against oxidative damage. Resveratrol, present in wine, gives further protection. Omega-3 fat in fish fights inflammation, known to be associated with risk for Alzheimer's disease. The antioxidant benefits of the diet translate into lower damage to the genes of learning and memory. The power molecules of the B vitamins and polyphenols (found in vegetables and fruit), resveratrol (found in wine), and omega-3 (found in fish) protect the genes of longevity in our brains.

EXERCISE MAKES YOU SMARTER

It is well known that a sedentary lifestyle increases the risk for cardiovascular disease, type 2 diabetes, osteoporosis, cancer, and depression. Conversely, an active lifestyle protects against these conditions. Physical exercise is crucial to protecting our brain. I know you have heard that walking can "clear your head." Aerobic exercise stimulates blood flow and oxygen delivery to the brain.

For many years it was thought that the brain cells you were born with were all that you would ever have. Dr. Fred Gage at the Salk Institute for Biological Studies in La Jolla, California, revolutionized neuroscience when he demonstrated this was not the case. Not only do we add new brain cells but the cells that are grown are located in the brain regions associated with memory and learning.

More recently, Dr. Gage has shown in studies with mice that we can encourage the development of new brain cells through physical exercise. It seems that brain cells are encouraged to grow by exercise. I think this makes perfect sense from an evolutionary perspective because active animals would be expected to be more alert to their surroundings to avoid danger.

Multitudes of studies have documented the benefits of aerobic exercise on the brain. Recent studies have shown protection against Parkinson's disease,[1] Alzheimer's dementia,[2] stroke,[3] and protection against falls caused by physical inactivity. Mood is elevated by exercise. Regular exercise has a beneficial effect on depression,[4] quality of sleep,[5] and cognitive function.[6] A recent study of fifty-nine healthy but sedentary individuals compared the effect of a walking program to a stretching/toning program, and MRIs showed an increase in brain volume in the brains of the aerobically exercising seniors after only six months.[7] No increase was noted for seniors in the stretch/tone group.

How does moving your muscles help your mind?

SYNAPTIC PRUNING

When we move our muscles we are activating pathways established in our youth when we first learned to walk, run, bike, play tennis, ski, ice skate, or whatever. If the pathways are not activated they fall into disuse, like an old trail that has not been traveled. Just as weeds grow over the trail, so that it is increasingly difficult to reach one's destination, so it is with these brain pathways. If we don't practice the skills, the paths are less defined in the brain. They are still there but finding them becomes difficult. The neurons of the brain communicate with one another by branching. If a neuron branch isn't used a process called *synaptic pruning* takes place. This means that old connections not being used are deleted. If you haven't ridden a bicycle since childhood and climb on as an adult, you still remember how to do it but you are shaky in your balance until the brain pathways are activated. So we need to keep practicing the skills that we have.

BRAIN PLASTICITY

Plasticity is your brain's way of forming new pathways when we learn and helps us to remember. It has been discovered that exercise increases the brain longevity molecules involved in learning and memory. Regular exercise increases the gene expression of brain growth factors (brain-derived neurotrophic factor and nerve-growth factor), making new pathways grow. Growth factors of the brain encourage plasticity. Most of the activity takes place in the very seat of memory, the brain hippocampus. It has been recently found that physical exercise increases the amount of brain growth in the hippocampus,[8] important for learning and memory.

We can encourage plasticity by learning new activities throughout our lives. Physically, learning a new skill like juggling is more challenging for a fifty-year-old than for a ten-year-old. But the physical act of juggling will encourage plasticity in your brain. You may be frustrated by the experience but the paths can be established and will benefit your most valuable asset, your mind. Learn a new dance—try the tango, salsa, hula—the steps that you learn are building paths in your brain! Exercise your body while you exercise your mind.

Specific ways of stimulating plasticity are activities that make you think. This means learning a new skill: how about the hula hoop, juggling, or using the skip-it ball? In my office, I ask the trainers to incorporate these activities into exercise routines. The idea is to stimulate your mind while exercising the body. One of the best ways to stimulate your mind and body is to learn a new dance or sport. Recently I was in Texas and had the pleasure of learning the Texas Two-Step; my husband and I laughed together and finally were able to perform the moves like we were born in the Lone Star State! We were clumsy at the beginning but now we know a new dance that we didn't know before! The moral of this story is to keep yourself open to new opportunities!

CONCLUSION

It is unfortunate that the U.S. diet revolves around overly processed foods high in sugar and fat. Vegetables are good for us but vegetable oils unnaturally overload the body with omega-6 fat. Corn and soybean oils and the sweetener corn syrup represent subsidized crops that keep snack food prices low. Diets high in these are simply not good for you. Nor are they good for the farmers who raise the crops or their children. This is the problem: The subsidized crops represent a livelihood for farm families. I am hopeful that we will replace the corn and soybean crops with healthier alternative crops soon. It is an enormously complex issue, but ignoring it will compound our already worsening obesity epidemic.

Our mayor in New York, Michael Bloomberg, has intervened on behalf of health in meaningful ways by banning smoking in restaurants, getting soda machines out of schools, and outlawing trans fats in restaurants. These interventions should encourage other politicians to change things. We need more of this.

But it is not only food that is robbing us of health and energy; our lives have become far too sedentary. Daily exercise is basic to life. Add exercise in every way possible: join a health club, hire a trainer, walk everywhere, and take the stairs at every opportunity. Exercise is like knowledge—its effect is cumulative.

Lifestyle has a tremendous effect on health. It matters enormously whether you exercise, eat properly, sleep adequately, and manage stress well. The exciting part is that we now know how these acts of daily life can cause changes within cells. Power molecules, which protect vegetables and fruits from damage from sunlight and insects, can protect our cells. Daily exercise causes new mitochondria and capillaries to form, resulting in a higher metabolism. Reaching the deepest stages of sleep allows for the production of growth hormone and leptin within the brain. Managing stress can influence the length of telomeres within the nucleus of the cell, a barometer of aging. The orchestration of the multitude of bodily processes is dependent on the choices we make. What we recognize as good health is a reflection of millions of small choices we make.

Your body is indeed wondrous. I sincerely hope that you will take care of yourself. It isn't even all that hard. Just start. Change habits that can harm your health and substitute habits that promote health. Every cell of your body and every neuron of your brain are worthy of your care. In this book I have outlined what I have seen work for others and I've given explanations of the physiology. People seem to do better when they know more, so I have explained mechanisms that underlie metabolism. The rest is up to you. Individuals change their lives all the time, and when it happens it inspires all of us.

I wish you well in your journey toward health and greater energy. You deserve the best.

CHAPTER ELEVEN

ENERGY EATING-PLAN RECIPES

BREAKFAST

Swiss Chard and Ricotta Omelet

Serves 1

 2 teaspoons extra virgin olive oil
 2 large omega-3 eggs
 ¼ cup cooked Swiss chard
 ¼ cup low-fat or fat-free ricotta cheese mixed with ¼ teaspoon
 cinnamon

1. Heat the oil in a small skillet.
2. Whisk together the eggs in a small bowl. Then add to the skillet.
3. Combine the Swiss chard and ricotta-cinnamon mixture.
4. When the eggs have set throughout, spread the cheese and Swiss chard mixture over them, and then fold over the omelet.

High-Energy Berry Blast

Serves 1

    ½ cup each blueberries, blackberries, and strawberries

    1 cup low-fat yogurt

    1 teaspoon ginger juice

    2 teaspoons honey

    2 teaspoons wheat germ

Put everything in a blender with 4 ice cubes. Puree until smooth. Serve in a tall glass.

Yogurt Energy Starter

Serves 1

    1 cup low-fat yogurt

    1 shot espresso

    ¼ cup fresh or frozen pitted sweet cherries

Put everything into a blender with 4 ice cubes. Puree until smooth. Serve in a tall glass.

Sunrise Chicken Quesadilla

Serves 1

    1 whole wheat tortilla

    2 tablespoons salsa

    3 ounces sliced leftover chicken

    ¼ cup sliced avocado

    2 ounces low-fat Jack or cheddar cheese, grated

    ¼ cup finely chopped papaya

1.   Put the tortilla on a plate and spread the salsa evenly over it. Arrange the chicken on top of the salsa. Top with the avocado and end with the grated cheese.

2. Put into the microwave oven until the cheese is melted.
3. Top with the chopped papaya. Serve.

Energy Omelet

Serves 1

    2 omega-3 eggs
    1 teaspoon reduced-fat or skim milk
    2 teaspoons olive oil
    2 ounces smoked salmon, cut into bite-size pieces
    ¼ cup cooked spinach
    Salt and pepper to taste
    Parsley (chopped for garnish)

1. Beat the eggs and the milk together.
2. Heat the oil in an omelet pan. When the oil is hot pour in the eggs, swirl them, and allow the bottom to set. Working with your spatula, keep the pan moving to cook the eggs through from the bottom.
3. When the egg is about halfway cooked, add the salmon and the spinach. Flip the omelet onto the other side, if necessary, or simply fold over and slip onto a plate.
4. Season with salt and pepper and garnish with parsley.

LUNCH OR DINNER

Ginger Soy Chicken

Serves 2

    2 boneless skinless chicken breasts, cut into ½-inch cubes
    2 tablespoons low-sodium soy sauce
    3 tablespoons ginger juice
    1 teaspoon rice wine vinegar
    1 to 2 tablespoons olive oil for stir-frying
    1 red pepper, cut into thin ½-inch slices
    1½ teaspoons freshly grated gingerroot
    3 chopped scallions
    ¼ cup chopped almonds

1. After washing and patting the chicken dry, marinate the chicken in soy sauce, ginger juice, and rice wine vinegar for 2 hours in the refrigerator.

2. Reserve the marinade. In a wok or large skillet, heat the oil and stir-fry the chicken and peppers separately at medium-high heat until tender. Remove the chicken and peppers from the pan and lower the heat to medium. Then add the fresh ginger and scallions to the wok and stir-fry for a few minutes.

3. Put the chicken and peppers back in the pan and stir-fry with the ginger and scallions. Add the reserved marinade and stir-fry for another minute.

4. Garnish with the chopped almonds and serve.

Spiced Shrimp with Cucumber Salad

Serves 4

I peeled cucumber, quartered lengthwise and cut into ½-inch slices

I small red onion, minced

I jalapeño chili pepper, seeded and minced

½ cup chopped fresh cilantro

I 7.75-ounce can hearts of palm, drained and sliced thin

Juice of I large orange (about ½ cup)

2 tablespoons balsamic vinegar

I½ pounds raw medium-sized shrimp, cleaned well

Pinch of coarse sea salt

Freshly ground black pepper to taste

I teaspoon cumin

½ teaspoon ground coriander

I tablespoon fresh chopped oregano

4 teaspoons olive oil

1. In a large bowl, toss together the cucumber, onion, jalapeño, hearts of palm, cilantro, orange juice, and vinegar. Season with the sea salt and pepper; set in the refrigerator for I hour.

2. Dust the shrimp with cumin, coriander, and oregano; season with the remaining ground pepper. In a large skillet, cook the 2 teaspoons of oil over high heat.

3. Cook the shrimp in three batches; do not crowd them. Brown both sides, 3 to 4 minutes. Transfer to a platter. Repeat until all the shrimp are done.
4. Remove the salad from the refrigerator. To serve, spoon the shrimp over the cucumber salad.

Salmon Croquettes

Serves 2

    1 6-ounce can of salmon, drained and flaked
    1 red pepper, chopped
    3 scallions, chopped
    ½ cup chopped parsley
    1 omega-3 egg
    ¼ cup wheat germ
    1 slice whole grain bread, grated into crumbs
    2 tablespoons canola oil in a skillet

1. Mix together the salmon, pepper, scallions, and parsley. In a separate bowl beat the egg. Then fold the egg into the salmon mixture.
2. Mix together the wheat germ and bread crumbs and combine the mixture with the salmon.
3. Form the salmon mixture into patties and brown in the oil for about 10 minutes, turning as the croquettes become brown.

Note: The croquettes can be made the size of burger patties or they can be small bite-size patties. It is an easy and healthful meal served over salad greens.

Selenium Salad

Serves 2

    2 tablespoons olive oil
    2 teaspoons balsamic vinegar
    Salad greens (I suggest 2 bunches of arugula)
    Dressing of extra virgin olive oil and balsamic vinegar
    2 tuna steaks, 1 inch thick
    Juice of 1 lemon

Zest of 1 lemon

2 Brazil nuts, slivered

1. Mix the olive oil and the balsamic vinegar together. Pour the mixture over the tuna and refrigerate for 3 hours.
2. Wash the salad greens and dry them. In a salad bowl, toss the greens with the dressing of olive oil and vinegar.
3. Grill the tuna over medium heat about 4 minutes on each side. (The tuna should not be overcooked.) Remove the steaks from heat and pour the lemon juice over them.
4. Arrange the salad on plates and place tuna on top of each salad. Top with lemon zest and slivered Brazil nuts.

Very Veggie Consommé

2 tablespoons olive oil

3 leeks, cut into ½-inch pieces

3 stalks celery, cut into ½-inch pieces

3 carrots, cut in half lengthwise, then into ½-inch pieces

1 medium zucchini cut into ½-inch circles

1 medium yellow squash, cut into ½-inch circles

1 Vidalia onion (any other kind works, but Vidalia is best) sliced

4 cloves unpeeled garlic

4 medium tomatoes, cored and cut in half

2 quarts water

1 handful parsley, roughly chopped

4 sprigs thyme

Kosher salt and freshly ground black pepper

1 bay leaf

1. Preheat the oven to 400°F.
2. In a roasting pan on top of the stove, heat the olive oil and brown the leeks, celery, carrots, zucchini, yellow squash, onion, and garlic. You want to just barely sear and singe the outside of the vegetables. This step should take only 5 minutes at most.
3. Add the tomatoes to the vegetables in the roasting pan, placing the toma-

toes with their cut sides down. Cover the pan and put in the oven for about 45 minutes. Stir the vegetables every 20 minutes or so. Don't let the vegetables burn, but do allow them to carmelize. The carmelizing process gives a robust flavor.

4. Bring 2 quarts of water to boil in a large pot. Add the roasted vegetables, scraping the brown bits from the bottom of the pan. Bring this to a simmer on top of the stove and add the parsley, thyme, and bay leaf. Cook for two hours gently.

5. Strain out the vegetables and reserve.

6. Boil down the liquid until it is concentrated and flavorful. This intensifies the flavor.

7. Puree the vegetables or press them through a food mill into the stock. Season to taste with salt and pepper.

White Bean and Escarole Soup

Serves 4

> 1 onion, chopped
> 2 cloves garlic, crushed
> 1 carrot, cut up
> 4 sprigs of fresh thyme
> ½ teaspoon coriander
> 2 tablespoons olive oil
> 1 head escarole, trimmed, washed, and coarsely chopped
> 4 cups of chicken broth (you can use Maggie Ella's recipe or a store-
>   bought brand of good quality)
> 2 15-ounce cans of cooked cannellini beans
> Kosher salt
> Freshly ground black pepper

1. In a soup pot, over a medium-high flame brown the onion, garlic, carrot, thyme, and coriander in olive oil. This takes just about 5 minutes or so. Stir in the escarole and cook until it is wilted.

2. Pour the chicken broth and the beans into the cooked vegetable mixture and bring to a simmer. Cook for 15 minutes. Do not overcook the beans!

3. Remove the thyme, if you like. Season to taste with salt and pepper.

DESSERTS

Dr. Klauer's Omega-3 Cake

Serves 6

   2 large omega-3 eggs
   ⅛ cup canola oil
   1½ cups 1 percent milk
   2 teaspoons baking powder
   3 teapoons pure vanilla extract
   ½ cup ground flaxseed
   ½ cup honey
   ¼ cup grated orange zest (about 3 large oranges)
   ¼ cup wheat germ
   ¼ cup pitted dried cherries
   ¾ cup chopped walnuts
   1 teaspoon ground ginger
   ½ teaspoon cinnamon
   ¼ teaspoon ground nutmeg
   2 cups whole wheat graham flour

1. Mix all ingredients thoroughly and pour into a pregreased 8 × 12-inch baking pan.
2. Bake for about 40 minutes at 325°F.
3. Cool slightly, cut into squares, and serve with berries and yogurt.

The following two recipes are from François Payard, owner of Payard Pâtisserie and Bistro. Both are delicious and surprisingly easy to make.

Pomegranate Granita

   1 7-ounce bottle pomegranate juice (POM)
   5 packets Splenda or Equal
   2 ounces water
   750 ml bottle pink champagne
   1 lemon, freshly squeezed

1. In a medium saucepan combine the pomegranate juice, Splenda, and water. Bring to a boil, puree, and then strain through a very fine sieve or cheesecloth. Add the champagne and the lemon juice to taste. Pour the mixture into a sheet pan and place in freezer.

2. Using a fork or serrated knife, scrape off the top crystallized layer as the granita freezes. Place the frozen scraped granita in a serving bowl or individual parfait cups. Each time a frozen layer is removed, return the sheet pan to the freezer and leave it there until the surface has frozen. Continue the process until all the mixture has been frozen and scraped.

3. Serve in pre-chilled parfait glasses.

Warm Raspberry Soufflé

Serves 6 to 8

You'll need a blender or food processor, an electric mixer fitted with the whip attachment, a pastry bag fitted with a round tip, and six to eight 4 cm diameter by 3 cm high ceramic ramekins.

Unsalted butter, room temperature
Sugar
2 pints fresh raspberries
4 egg yolks
4 packets Splenda or Equal for the yolks
10 egg whites, room temperature
½ lemon, juiced
1 tablespoon cornstarch to stabilize the egg whites

1. Preheat the oven to 170°F. Butter the insides of the molds using a pastry brush and chill them for 15 minutes. Brush them again with the butter and coat the insides with sugar. Pour out any excess sugar and reserve the molds in the refrigerator.

2. Combine fresh raspberries, egg yolks, and Splenda in a blender and blend for several minutes to emulsify. Place the raspberry mixture in a medium-size bowl.

3. Place the egg whites into the bowl of an electric mixer fitted with the whip attachment and whip on slow speed. When the whites are foamy, add the lemon juice and whisk on medium speed until they form soft

peaks. Add the cornstarch. Fold one scoop of the meringue into the raspberry mixture. Gently fold in the rest of the meringue.

4. Fill a pastry bag fitted with a large round tip with the soufflé mixture. Fill each mold ¾ full. Using your thumb, wipe the edge of the mold to remove any excess soufflé mixture and the sugar and butter from the rim. Bake the soufflés in the oven for 8 minutes for a moist center or 10 minutes for a firmer and center. Remove the soufflés from the oven and serve immediately.

Note: The secret to high, stable soufflés is to separate the eggs the night before and leave the whites out overnight. Room-temperature egg whites whip firmer and to a larger volume than cold whites.

L and C's Famous Zucchini Bread
From Susan Allport, author of *The Queen of Fats*

Makes 2 small loaves

3 omega-3 eggs
2 cups sugar
2 cups grated zucchini
1 cup canola oil
2 cups flour
¼ teaspoons baking powder
¼ teaspoon baking soda
1 teaspoon salt
3 teaspoons cinnamon
1 cup chopped walnuts
3 teaspoons vanilla

Beat the eggs and add the sugar, zucchini, and oil. Mix well. Sift all the dry ingredients except the walnuts together and add to the egg mixture. Add the nuts and vanilla. Bake in a greased pan at 350°F for 75 minutes.

From Susan Allport: My daughters made their reputations as bakers with this tasty bread. It's our favorite way of using excess zucchini, and it freezes well. The zucchini, eggs, walnuts, and canola oil are all sources of omega-3s.

STARTERS, DRESSINGS, AND SIDES

Great Grapes Dressing

Makes about 3 cups

  2 cups red wine
  1 bay leaf
  ¼ cup red wine vinegar
  1 tablespoon Dijon mustard
  ½ teaspoon salt
  ½ teaspoon freshly ground pepper
  2 cups grapeseed oil

1. In a medium saucepan, bring wine and bay leaf to a boil. Reduce the heat to simmer, stirring occasionally for about 10 minutes or until reduced by half.
2. Remove and discard the bay leaf.
3. Combine the reduced wine mixture, mustard, salt, and pepper in a blender. Process until smooth. Gradually add the oil. Store in the refrigerator.

This is also a great marinade for fish and veggies on the grill.

Ginger Lemonade

Serves 4
  1 large bottle San Pellegrino
  4 tablespoons freshly squeezed lemon juice
  2 tablespoons ginger juice*
  Honey or Splenda if desired, sweeten to taste
  1 mint sprig, for garnish

Mix, garnish with a sprig of mint, and serve over ice in a tall glass.

*Ginger juice can be found in Whole Foods Markets or at www.gingerpeople .com

Roasted Sweet Potato Fries

Serves 4

    2 large unpeeled sweet potatoes
    1½ teaspoons ground cumin
    1 teaspoon ground coriander
    ½ teaspoon freshly ground pepper
    1 tablespoon olive oil
    Coarse salt to taste

1. Scrub the potatoes. Cut them in half lengthwise and then into thin strips, or use a french fry cutter.
2. In a bowl, mix together the cumin, coriander, and ground pepper. Add the olive oil.
3. Toss the potatoes with olive oil and spices in a large plastic bag or in a bowl.
4. On a baking sheet coated with nonstick spray, bake the potatoes in a 400°F preheated oven for 20 minutes. Turn and bake on the other side for 10 minutes. The fries should be brown and crisp.
5. Toss with coarse salt.

Stella's Dandelion Greens

Serves 4

    1 clove garlic (crushed)
    1 tablespoon olive oil
    5 cups washed dandelion greens
    Juice of one medium lemon

1. In a frying pan over medium heat cook the garlic in the oil until the garlic is just translucent.
2. Add the dandelions, stirring them gently as the olive oil coats their leaves.
3. Cover with lid just for 30 seconds to allow the steam to penetrate the leaves.
4. Toss with lemon and serve.

Spring Salad with Purslane and Baby Spinach

Serves 2
  Salad
  2 cups purslane, washed and torn into pieces
  2 cups baby spinach, washed and torn into pieces
  1 cup sliced baby strawberries, washed and sliced
  Dressing
  1 tablespoon extra virgin olive oil
  2 teaspoons raspberry vinegar
  2 teaspoons cherry juice
  1 teaspoon dry mustard

Mix all the dressing ingredients together. Toss the dressing into salad, but avoid overdressing the greens.

Maggie Ella's Good-for-You Chicken Soup

My grandmother always seemed to have a pot of soup simmering on the stove. The reason for this was she used the bones leftover from meals, wilting herbs and vegetables to make her delicious soup. She just tossed everything into the soup pot without ever looking at a cookbook. As an experienced cook, she could get away with this. You can modify her thrifty method by saving bones from chicken and turkey meals in a large Ziploc bag in your freezer. When you have a large collection throw everything into a soup pot. The different types of bones make the broth extra rich.

   The version that I present here is my adaptation of her soup.

  1 cut-up chicken
  4 stalks chopped celery
  4 chopped carrots
  1 onion, peeled and studded with 10 cloves
  1 bay leaf
  A handful of parsley sprigs, thyme sprigs, and basil

1. Put the chicken and the vegetables in a large soup pot and cover with about one inch of water. Bring the broth to a boil.

2. When water is boiling, skim the scum off the top. Reduce the heat so that the broth is just simmering, cover the pot partially, and continue to skim off the scum every few minutes. Cook for about one hour.

3. After one hour, remove the chicken to a platter, take off the skin, and remove all bones. Cut the chicken into 1-inch cubes and set aside and discard all the skin.

4. Strain out the vegetables and herbs, then puree them in a food mill or with a food processor, and put the mixture back into the soup. Add the cubed chicken. Taste the broth, season with salt and pepper, and refrigerate.

5. After refrigeration fat will accumulate at the top of the broth and should be removed with a spoon. Prior to serving, bring the soup to a boil and add 2 cups of a leafy vegetable such as spinach, watercress, or escarole. Cook for a few minutes, taste, adjust seasonings, and serve.

APPENDIX

NUTRITIONAL COMPONENTS OF GRAIN

GRAIN	WHAT IT IS	NUTRITIONAL INFORMATION
Amaranth ¼ cup dry	Amaranth provides protein, calcium, iron, and zinc. The protein and iron content and concentration of the amino acids lysine and methionine are higher than in many grains.	Calories = 182 Total Fat = 3.25g Saturated Fat = 0.75g Cholesterol = 0mg Sodium = 10.25mg Carbohydrate = 32.25g Dietary Fiber = 4.5g Protein = 4g
Barley ¼ cup dry	Barley is an excellent ingredient for providing soluble fiber, and is rich in niacin and iron. Whole	Calories = 163 Total Fat = 1g Saturated Fat = 0.25g Cholesterol = 0mg

Nutritional Components of Grain

GRAIN	WHAT IT IS	NUTRITIONAL INFORMATION
	barley, also called hulled barley (the inedible husk has been removed), is more nutritious than pearled barley because the bran is left intact.	Sodium = 5.5mg Carbohydrate = 33.75g Dietary Fiber = 8g Protein = 5.75g
Buckwheat ¼ cup dry	Buckwheat is a rich source of the amino acid lysine. It contains high levels of protein, calcium, magnesium, phosphorous, B vitamins, and iron. Because it contains no gluten, buckwheat is a good wheat substitute for people who are allergic to gluten.	Calories = 146 Total Fat = 1.5g Saturated Fat = 0.25g Cholesterol = 0mg Sodium = 0.5mg Carbohydrate = 30.5g Dietary Fiber = 4.25g Protein = 5.75g
Corn ¼ cup dry	Corn is a good source of vitamin A, manganese, and potassium. It contains protein, but it is not a particularly good source. Many other grains contain a greater ratio of protein than corn.	Calories = 152 Total Fat = 2g Saturated Fat = 0.25g Cholesterol = 0mg Sodium = 14.5mg Carbohydrate = 30.75g Dietary Fiber = 3g Protein = 4g
Flaxseed ¼ cup dry	Flaxseed is one of the best sources of omega-3 fatty acids. The seeds contain soluble fiber, which also helps in reducing cholesterol	Calories = 224 Total Fat = 17.75g Saturated Fat = 1.5g Cholesterol = 0mg Sodium = 12.5mg

Nutritional Components of Grain

GRAIN	WHAT IT IS	NUTRITIONAL INFORMATION
	levels. About one third of the fiber in flaxseed is soluble and two-thirds is insoluble, which is an important component in aiding digestion. Flaxseed is the best source of lignin, which may play a role in fighting certain types of cancer.	Carbohydrate = 12.25g Dietary Fiber = 11.5g Protein = 7.75g
Millet ¼ cup dry	Millet is an excellent source of iron and magnesium and is also high in calcium, phosphorous, manganese, zinc, and B vitamins. It has the highest iron content of any grain except amaranth and quinoa. The natural alkalinity of millet makes it easily digestible, so it is very beneficial for people with ulcers and digestive problems, and is one of the least allergenic of all grains.	Calories = 189 Total Fat = 2g Saturated Fat = 0.25g Cholesterol = 0mg Sodium = 2.5mg Carbohydrate = 36.5g Dietary Fiber = 4.25g Protein = 5.5g
Oats ¼ cup dry	Oats are one of the most nutritious grains and a good source of the soluble fiber beta-glucan, which helps to decrease cholesterol in the blood. Other important nutrients found in oats are B vitamins, vitamin E,	Calories = 152 Total Fat = 2.75g Saturated Fat = 0.5g Cholesterol = 0mg Sodium = 0.75mg Carbohydrate = 25.75g Dietary Fiber = 4.25g Protein = 6.5g

NUTRITIONAL COMPONENTS OF GRAIN

GRAIN	WHAT IT IS	NUTRITIONAL INFORMATION
	copper, iron, zinc, magnesium, phosphorous, calcium, and thiamin.	
Quinoa ¼ cup dry	Nutritionally, quinoa is an excellent grain. It is loaded with protein and the amino acid lysine. It contains about 17 percent high-quality protein, which is more than any other grain and is equivalent to milk in protein quality. Quinoa is also very high in iron and is an important source of calcium, zinc, potassium, magnesium, phosphorus, and copper.	Calories = 159 Total Fat = 2.5g Saturated Fat = 0.25g Cholesterol = 0mg Sodium = 9mg Carbohydrate = 29.25g Dietary Fiber = 2.5g Protein = 5.5g
Rice ¼ cup dry	White rice has had the husk, bran, and germ removed, which allows it to cook rapidly. This makes it the least nutritious grain because of the removal of the bran and germ. White rice is often enriched with nutrients, such as iron, niacin, thiamin, and riboflavin (especially in Western nations), to help restore some of the lost nutritional value. Flour milled from rice contains no	Calories = 171 Total Fat = 1.75g Saturated Fat = 0.25g Cholesterol = 0mg Sodium = 3.25mg Carbohydrate = 35.75g Dietary Fiber = 1.5g Protein = 3.75g

Nutritional Components of Grain

GRAIN	WHAT IT IS	NUTRITIONAL INFORMATION
	gluten so it is an excellent choice for people who are gluten-intolerant.	
Rye ¼ cup dry	Rye is an excellent source of dietary fiber as well as vitamin E, calcium, iron, thiamin, phosphorus, and potassium.	Calories = 142 Total Fat = 1g Saturated Fat = 0g Cholesterol = 0mg Sodium = 2.5mg Carbohydrate = 29.5g Dietary Fiber = 6.25g Protein = 6.25g
Sorghum ¼ cup dry	Nutritionally, sorghum is similar to corn, but it has a higher concentration of protein. It lacks gluten so it is an excellent choice for people who are gluten-intolerant.	Calories = 163 Total Fat = 1.5g Saturated Fat = 0.25g Cholesterol = 0mg Sodium = 3mg Carbohydrate = 33.75g Dietary Fiber = 3g Protein = 5.5g
Spelt ¼ cup dry	Spelt is making a comeback in the United States not only because of its good flavor, but also because of its nutritional qualities. Spelt contains a higher level of protein (up to 25 percent more) than soft white wheat varieties, but it has a protein level that is the	Calories = 140 Total Fat = 1g Saturated Fat = 0.25g Cholesterol = 0mg Sodium = 0mg Carbohydrate = 31g Dietary Fiber = 3g Protein = 6g

GRAIN	WHAT IT IS	NUTRITIONAL INFORMATION
	same or less than hard red wheat varieties. It is a rich source of B vitamins and fiber. Other nutrients found in spelt include iron, magnesium, niacin, thiamin, and phosphorus. It has been shown that the carbohydrate in spelt are useful in enhancing the immune system and in helping to clot the blood.	
Teff ¼ cup dry	Because the teff grain is so small, there is no way to remove the husk, bran, and germ, which means that none of the nutrients are lost as is the case with larger grains that have had the bran and germ removed during processing. Teff is high in calcium, iron, magnesium, zinc, and thiamin, and it is a good source of fiber.	Calories = 160 Total Fat = 1g Saturated Fat = 0g Cholesterol = 0mg Sodium = 10mg Carbohydrate = 33g Dietary Fiber = 6g Protein = 6g
Triticale ¼ cup dry	Triticale combines the nutritional benefits of both wheat and rye. It has a high-protein content and it also contains a high level of lysine that is common in rye. There is a greater quantity of folic	Calories = 161 Total Fat = 1g Saturated Fat = 0.25g Cholesterol = 0mg Sodium = 2.5mg Carbohydrate = 34.5g Dietary Fiber = 0g

NUTRITIONAL COMPONENTS OF GRAIN

GRAIN	WHAT IT IS	NUTRITIONAL INFORMATION
	acid, pantothenic acid, copper, and vitamin B_6 in triticale than in wheat, but a lesser quantity of niacin. Triticale is also an important source of iron, thiamin, magnesium, phosphorus, potassium, zinc, and it is rich in fiber.	Protein = 6.25g
Wheat ¼ cup dry	Among the nutrients present in whole wheat are high levels of protein, fiber, iron, B vitamins, thiamin, niacin, magnesium, phosphorus, and zinc. Studies have shown that the insoluble fiber in wheat bran may help fight colon cancer and at the very least is beneficial for the digestion.	Calories = 158 Total Fat = 1g Saturated Fat = 0.25g Cholesterol = 0mg Sodium = 1mg Carbohydrate = 32.75g Dietary Fiber = 5.75g Protein = 7.5g
Wild Rice ¼ cup dry	Wild rice is one of the most nutritious grainlike foods. It is very low in fat and very high in fiber. In addition, it has nearly twice the protein of true rice varieties and it is loaded with B vitamins, folate, niacin, thiamin, iron, phosphorus, zinc, and magnesium.	Calories = 143 Total Fat = 0.5g Saturated Fat = 0g Cholesterol = 0mg Sodium = 2.75mg Carbohydrate = 30g Dietary Fiber = 2.5g Protein = 6g

Source: www.recipetips.com

Glycemic Index for Carbohydrate

FRESH FRUITS	GI	VEGETABLES	GI	GRAINS	GI
Cherry	22	Artichoke	0	Barley (pearl)	25
Grapefruit	25	Avocado	0	Barley	43
Apple	38	Broccoli (raw)	0	Cracked Wheat (bulgur)	48
Pear	38	Lettuce	0	Buckwheat	54
Plum	39	Cucumber	0	Oat Bran (raw)	55
Strawberry	40	Peppers	0	Couscous (cooked)	65
Orange	42	Celery	0	Cornmeal	69
Peach	42	Spinach	0	Millet (cooked)	71
Grape	46	Cauliflower	0		
Mango	51	Cabbage (raw)	0		
Banana	51	Squash (raw)	0		
Kiwi	53	Yam	37		
Apricot	57	Carrots (raw)	47		
Pineapple	59	Green Peas	48		
Cantaloupe	65	Sweet Corn (cooked)	54		
Watermelon	72	Beet	64		
		Pumpkin	75		

Source: www.carbs-information.com

HEALTHY EATING

RESOURCES

http://intl-jcem.endojournals.org
  The Journal of Clinical Endocrinology and Metabolism.
www.aafp.org/online/en/home.html
  The home page for the American Academy of Family Physicians.
www.aicr.org
  The home page for the America Institute for Cancer Research.
http://content.nejm.org
  The home page for the *New England Journal of Medicine.*
www.nih.gov
  The home page for the National Institutes of Health. You can calculate your body
mass index at http://www.nhlbisupport.com/bmi/.
http://jama.ama-assn.org
  The American Medical Association and *JAMA* home page.
www.mayoclinic.com
  The Mayo Clinic's home page.
www.fda.gov
  The official Web site for the Food and Drug Administration.
www.nlm.nih.gov/medlineplus
  A consumer site that brings together information from the National Library of

Medicine (NLM), the National Institutes of Health (NIH), and other government and health-related organizations.

www.eatright.org

The American Dietetic Association site has resources for up-to-date information on food and nutrition.

http://www.mypyramid.gov

The new 2005 food pyramid from the U.S. Department of Agriculture.

www.nutritiondata.com

This contains complete nutrition information: facts, tools, and recipes.

VEGETARIANS

www.vrg.org

The Vegetarian Resource Group, a nonprofit organization dedicated to educating the public on vegetarianism, health, and nutrition. Includes a guide to natural foods restaurants in the United States and Canada.

www.nutrition.gov

A resource list for vegetarians from the Food and Nutrition Information Center.

www.veggieglobal.com

A portal for vegetarians with links, recipes, support groups, and resources worldwide.

KIDS AND TEENS

www.42explore.com/eggs.htm

42explore contains basic information on eggs with activities and Web quests.

www.5aday.com

The site, 5 a day the color way, eat your colors, emphasizes the colors of health as blue/purple, green, white, yellow/orange, and red—the colors of fruit and vegetables.

http://aggie-horticulture.tamu.edu/nutrition

The site gives information on the relationship between gardens and healthy eating geared toward upper elementary students.

http://library.thinkquest.org/10991

This is a site created by students on nutrition for teens.

www.coolfoodplanet.org/gb/adoz/index.htm

The Web site, cool food adoz (adolescents), is a lively page for adolescents on healthy eating habits.

www.eatsmart.org

The Web site of the Washington State Dairy Council.

New York's Energy-Boosting Restaurants

These are some of my favorite restaurants to recommend to my patients, where healthy eating is a way of life and energizing meals abound!

Payard Patisserie & Bistro

The restaurant's elegant belle époque interior and warm hospitality create the right environment for enjoying the wondrous food. Chef and owner François Payard creates the most beautiful desserts in New York City.

1032 Lexington Avenue (between Seventy-third and Seventy-fourth Streets)

212-717-5252

www.payard.com

Blue Hill at Stone Barns

The former carriage house of the Rockefeller estate now houses a restaurant run by chef Dan Barber. And what a restaurant it is! Vegetables are grown in carefully tended rows on the property, chickens in immaculate coops supply the eggs, and all the food is deliciously organic. The restaurant is a forty-minute drive from New York City.

630 Bedford Road

Pocantico Hills, N.Y. 10591

914-366-9600

www.bluehillstonebarns.com

Blue Hill Restaurant

A Washington Square garden spot with innovative organic cuisine.

75 Washington Place

212-539-1776

www.bluehillnyc.com

Davidburke & Donatella

Fresh, creatively prepared cuisine.

133 East Sixty-first Street (between Park and Lexington)

212-813-2121

www.dbdrestaurant.com

Le Bilboquet

This tiny restaurant is so chic there is no name outside. Delicious salads and fish; the cajun chicken is very tasty.

　25 East Sixty-third Street (between Madison and Park)

　212-308-1659

HEALTHY MEALS AND SNACKS

Pret à Manger

The Euro chain that has hit it big in New York. These are healthier fast food–style places; just watch the calories on some of their prepared foods. www.pret.com/us

Hale & Hearty

Great for soups, salads, and crunchy sandwiches, with ten locations citywide.

　www.haleandhearty.com

Josie's

Vegetarian fare and wholesome foods.

　www.josiesnyc.com

Better Burger

Alternative fast food chain with air-baked fries and lighter burgers.

　www.betterburgernyc.com

Citarella to Go

A branch of the gourmet market, this takeout location near Radio City Music Hall is a winner.

　www.citarella.com

Marché Madison

A casual minimart of fine foods with a small counter for food on the run.

CASUAL EATING

Odeon
Tribeca classic Franco-American brasserie.
www.theodeonrestaurant.com

La Goulue
Uptown spot for ladies who lunch offering great salads in a Euro atmosphere.
www.lagouluerestaurant.com

Spring Street Natural
Neighborhood cozy place for crunchy, healthy food. Great for brunch.
www.springstreetnatural.com

The Pump
Low-fat and high-protein offerings for the gym crowd.
www.thepumpenergyfood.com

GREAT BREAKFASTS

Sarabeth's
Famous New York preppie breakfast and brunch spots with egg-white fritattas
served to your taste. Just say no to the oversized muffins.
www.sarabeths.com

Norma's
In the Parker Meridien, this yummy new American restaurant is a hot spot for
diners in search of something different.
www.parkermeridien.com

Fives at the Peninsula Hotel
Mediterranean-inspired fresh cuisine in a luxurious setting.
www.peninsula.com

ELEGANT DINING

Aquavit
Serves fresh salmon and herring a million ways.
www.aquavit.org

Park Avenue Autumn
The name and menu change with the seasons.
www.parkavenyc.com

Wild Salmon
A Midtown seafood favorite, with salmon flown in from the Pacific Northwest.
www.chinagrillmgt.com

Nobu
Pricey sushi for the tony banker crowd; exquisite presentation, and portions well under control.
www.myriadrestaurantgroup.com

Daniel
Is there anyone who has not heard of Daniel Boulud? His elegant restaurant offers French food in high style.
www.danielnyc.com

VEGAN AND VEGETARIAN CHOICES

Pure Food and Wine
Gramercy Park location with delicious vegan/vegetarian menu.
www.purefoodandwine.com

Tossed
Dubbed a "rabbit heaven," it offers healthy salad options with two popular Midtown locations.
www.tossed.com

Blossom Gourmet Vegetarian

Stylish Chelsea vegetarian and vegan dining.

www.blossomnyc.com

Gobo

Two locations with tasty and flavorful vegetarian dishes.

www.goborestaurant.com

ENERGIZING FOODS RESOURCES

Stonyfield Farms Yogurt

www.stonyfieldfarms.com

Fishing Vessel St. Jude Canned Albacore Tuna

www.tunatuna.com

Organic Valley

www.organicvalley.com

Fage

www.fage.com

Gnu Bar

www.gnufoods.com

Lärabar

www.larabar.com

Kashi

www.kashi.com

Eden Organics

www.edenfoods.com

Whole Foods

www.wholefoodsmarket.com

Trader Joe's

www.traderjoes.com

Fresh Direct

www.freshdirect.com

Peapod

www.peapod.com

Grace's Marketplace

www.gracesmarketplace.com

EVERYDAY NUTRITION

ENERGY JOURNAL

DATE _____

DAILY GOAL

_____

_____

_____

SLEEP

BEDTIME _____   AWAKENING _____

EXERCISE

ACTIVITY / DURATION _____

MEALS

Don't allow more than four hours to elapse between each meal and your snack.
Be sure to include protein.

TIME _____   BREAKFAST _____

TIME _____   LUNCH _____

TIME _____   AFTERNOON SNACK _____

TIME _____   DINNER _____

TIME _____   BEDTIME _____

GLASSES OF WATER _____   ALCOHOL _____

RECOMMENDED READING

For those who wish to read more about ways to become energetic, I suggest the following three books:

The Queen of Fats by Susan Allport

Everyone should read her well-written book on the role of omega-3 fat for our health.

Train Your Mind, Change Your Brain by Sharon Begley

The book outlines the neuroscience behind the ability of the mind to change the brain.

Younger Next Year by Chris Crowley and Henry S. Lodge, M.D.

The authors are on a mission to encourage the whole world to exercise daily.

NOTES

2. Three Bad Habits and How to Break Them

1. Chi-Tang Ho, et al., "Link Between Diabetes and High Fructose Corn Syrup," reported at the 234th national meeting of the American Chemical Society (2007).

2. Richard J. Johnson, et al., "Potential Role of Sugar (Fructose) in the Epidemic of Hypertension, Obesity and the Metabolic Syndrome, Diabetes, Kidney Disease and Cardiovascular Disease," *The American Journal of Clinical Nutrition* 86, no. 4 (October 2006): 899–906.

3. Energy Boosters: Omega-3, Protein, and Calcium

1. Chris Crowley and Henry S. Lodge, M.D., www.youngernextyear.com (accessed March 5, 2008).

2. Agricultural Health Study. www.aghealth.org/background.html (accessed January 25, 2008).

4. Energy Busters: Sugar, Sugar, Sugar!

1. Rob M. van Dam and Frank B. Hu, "Coffee Consumption and Risk of Type 2 Diabetes," *Journal of the American Medical Association* 294, no. 1 (July 6, 2005): 97–104.

5. Everyday Energy Plan

1. Fulvio Lauretani, Richard D. Semba, Stefania Bandinelli, et al., "Association of Low Plasma Selenium Concentration with Poor Muscle Strength in Community-Dwelling Adults: the InCHIANTI Study," *The American Journal of Clinical Nutrition* 86, no. 2 (August 2007): 347–52.

6. Power Molecules in Food

1. Barbara J. Lyle, Julie A. Mares-Perlman, Barbara E. K. Klein, et al., "Antioxidant Intake and Risk of Incident Age-Related Nuclear Cataracts in the Beaver Dam Eye Study," *The American Journal of Epidemiology* 149, no. 9 (May 1999): 801–809.
2. Lisa Chasan-Taber, Walter C. Willett, Johanna M. Seddon, et al., "A Prospective Study of Carotenoid and Vitamin A Intakes and Risk of Cataract Extraction in U.S. Women," *The American Journal of Clinical Nutrition* 70, no. 4 (October 1999): 509–16.
3. Julie A. Marse-Perlman, Alicia I. Fisher, Ronald Klein, et al., "Lutein and Zeax-anthin in the Diet and Serum and Their Relation to Age-Related Maculopathy in the Third National Health and Nutrition Examination Survey," *The American Journal of Epidemiology* 153, no. 5 (March 2001): 424–32.
4. Manoharan Shunmugam and Augusto Azuara-Blanco, "The Quality of Report-ing of Diagnostic Accuracy Studies in Glaucoma Using the Heidelberg Retina Tomograph," *Investigative Ophthalmology and Visual Science* 47, no. 6 (June 2006): 2317–23.
5. Claudine Manach, Augustin Scalbert, Christian Rémésy, and Liliana Jiménez, "Polyphenols: Food Sources and Bioavailability," *The American Journal of Clinical Nutrition* 79, no. 5 (March 2004): 727–47.
6. U.S.D.A. Agricultural Research Service. www.ars.usda.gov/nutrientdata (ac-cessed January 29, 2008).
7. Paul R. Thomas and Robert Earl, eds. *Opportunities in the Nutrition and Food Sciences: Research Challenges and the Next Generation of Investigators* (Washington, D.C.: The Na-tional Academy Press, 1994), 109.
8. Niamh O'Kennedy, Lynn Crosbie, Stuart Whelan, et al., "Effects of Tomato Ex-tract on Platelet Function: A Double-Blinded Crossover Study in Healthy Hu-mans," *The American Journal of Clinical Nutrition* 84, no. 3 (September 2006): 561–69.
9. Bente L. Halvorsen, Monica H. Carlsen, Katherine M. Phillips, et al., "Content of Redox-Active Compounds (i.e., Antioxidants) in Foods Consumed in the United States," *The American Journal of Clinical Nutrition* 84, no. 1 (July 2006): 95–135.
10. Ibid.

7. Omega-3: King of Land and Sea

1. GISSI Prevenzione Investigators, "Dietary Supplementation with N-3 Polyun-saturated Fatty Acids and Vitamin E After Myocardial Infarction, Results of the GISSI-Prevenzione Trial," *The Lancet* 354, no. 9177 (August 1999): 447–455.

2. Mitsuhiro Yokoyama et al., "Effects of Eicosapentaenoic Acid on Major Coronary Events in Hypercholesterolemic Patients (JELLIS): A Randomized, Open-Label, Blinded Endpoint Analysis," *The Lancet* 369, no. 9567 (March 31, 2007): 1090–8.

3. David Fryxell, "Special Report: Studies Find New Omega-3 Benefits," Tufts University Health & Nutrition Letter (July 2007).

4. A. P. Simopoulos, "The Role of Fatty Acids in Gene Expression: Health Implications," *Annals of Nutrition and Metabolism* 40, no. 6 (1996): 303–11.

5. Jagveer Singh, Rachid Hamid, and Bandaru S. Reddy, "Dietary Fat and Colon Cancer: Modulating Effect of Types and Amount of Dietary Fat on *ras*-p21 Function During Promotion and Progression Stages of Colon Cancer," *Cancer Research* 57, no. 2 (January 1997): 253–58.

8. The Energy Workout

1. Roberta Rikli, C. Jessie Jones. *Senior Fitness Test Manual* (Champaign, Ill.: Human Kinetics, 2001), 161.

2. R. Bohannon, P. Larkin, A. Cook, et al. "Decrease in Timed Balance Test Scores with Aging," *Physical Therapy* 64, no. 7 (July 1984): 1067–70.

3. Adapted and modified from *The Canadian Physical Activity, Fitness and Lifestyle Approach: CSEP-Health and Fitness Program's Health-Related Appraisal and Counseling Strategy*, 3rd ed. (Ottawa: Canadian Society for Exercise Physiology, 2003).

4. Ibid., and from *ACSM's Guidelines for Exercise Testing and Prescription*, 7th ed. (Indianapolis: American College of Sports Medicine, 2007).

5. Modified and adapted from the *YMCA Fitness Testing and Assessment Manual* (Champaign, Ill.: Human Kinetics, 1989).

9. The Sleep Factor

1. Wayne Hening, Arthur S. Walters, Richard P. Allen, et al., "Impact, Diagnosis and Treatment of Restless Legs Syndrome (RLS) in a Primary Care Population: The REST (RLS Epidemiology, Symptoms, and Treatment) Primary Care Study," *Sleep Medicine* 5, no. 3 (May 2004): 237–46.

10. Live Longer, Look Younger

1. Amanda D. Smith and Michael J. Zigmond, "Can the Brain Be Protected Through Exercise? Lessons from an Animal Model of Parkinsonism," *Experimental Neurology* 184, no. 1 (November 2003): 31–39.

2. C. W. Cotman and N. C. Berchtold, "Exercise: A Behavioral Intervention to Enhance Brain Health and Plasticity," *Trends in Neuroscience* 25, no. 6 (June 2002): 295–301.

3. W. Stummer, K. Weber, B. Tranmer, et al., "Reduced Mortality and Brain Damage After Locomotor Activity in Gerbil Forebrain Ischemia," *Stroke* 25, no. 9 (September 1994): 1862–69.

4. James A. Blumenthal, Michael A. Babyak, Kathleen A. Moore, et al., "Effects of Exercise Training on Older Patients with Major Depression," *Archives of Internal Medicine* 159, no. 19 (1999): 2349–59.

5. H. S. Driver and S. R. Taylor, "Exercise and Sleep," *Sleepmedicine Review,* 4, no. 4 (August 2000): 387–402.

6. Stanley J. Colcombe, Arthur F. Kramer, Kirk I. Erickson, et al., "Cardiovascular Fitness, Cortical Plasticity, and Aging," *Proceedings of the National Academy of Science* 101, no. 9 (March 2004): 3316–21.

7. Stanley K. Colcombe, Kirk I. Erickson, et al., "Aerobic Exercise Training Increases Brain Volume in Aging Humans," *The Journals of Gerontology Series A: Biological Sciences and Medical Sciences* 61 (2006): 1166–70.

8. Shoshanna Vaynman, Zhe Ying, and Fernando Gomez-Pinilla, "Hippocampal BDNF Mediates the Efficacy of Exercise on Synaptic and Cognition," *European Journal Neuroscience* 20, no. 10 (November 2004): 2580–90.

INDEX

Entries in small capitals indicate recipes.

EVERYDAY NUTRITION ORDER FORM

Send to:

Healthy Interventions

780 Park Avenue

New York, N.Y. 10021

If you'd like to order online, visit www.janaklauermd.com/products.aspx.

QUANTITY

_____ **Rich Cocoa** $114 per case of 24

The cocoa shake is from the highest-quality Brazilian cocoa beans. Cocoa naturally contains theobromine, a compound that makes us feel pleasure.

_____ **Vanilla Bean** $114 per case of 24

Dr. Klauer's Ready-to-Drink Meal Replacement Vanilla Bean Shake. The vanilla shake is delicious without an overly sweet taste.

_____ Subtotal

_____ Sales Tax (8.375% in New York)

_____ Shipping

_____ **Total**

PAYMENT METHOD

_____ Check   _____ Credit Card

                         _____ Expiration Date

_____

Signature

_____

Name

_____

Address

_____

City   State   Zip

_____

Phone number

_____

E-mail address